Transfer Boy

Perspectives on Asperger Syndrome

Ljiljana Vuletic,
Michel Ferrari
and Teodor Mihail

Jessica Kingsley Publishers
London and Philadelphia

Extracts on p.107, p.110, p.112, p.135, p.138, p.177 from Barron, J. and Barron, S. (2002) *There's a Boy in Here.* Arlington, TX: Future Horizons. Reproduced with kind permission.

First published in 2005
by Jessica Kingsley Publishers
116 Pentonville Road
London N1 9JB, UK
and
400 Market Street, Suite 400
Philadelphia, PA 19106, USA

www.jkp.com

Library of Congress Cataloging in Publication Data

Vuletic, Ljiljana, 1959-
Transfer boy : perspectives on Asperger syndrome / Ljiljana Vuletic, Michel Ferrari and Teodor Mihail.
p. cm.
Includes bibliographical references and index.
ISBN 1-84310-213-7 (pbk.)
1. Mihail, Teodor—Mental health. 2. Asperger's syndrome—Case studies. I. Ferrari, M.V.P. II. Mihail, Teodor. III. Title.
RJ506.A9V84 2005
616.85'88—dc22

2004020734

British Library Cataloguing in Publication Data

A CIP catalogue record for this book is available from the British Library

ISBN-13: 978 184310 213 7
ISBN-10: 1 84310 213 7

Printed and Bound in Great Britain by
Athenaeum Press, Gateshead, Tyne and Wear

Transfer Boy

of related interest

Asperger's Syndrome
A Guide for Parents and Professionals
Tony Attwood
Foreword by Lorna Wing
ISBN 1 85302 577 1

Asperger Syndrome, Adolescence, and Identity
Looking Beyond the Label
Harvey Molloy and Latika Vasil
ISBN 1 84310 126 2

Asperger Syndrome and Psychotherapy
Understanding Asperger Perspectives
Paula Jacobsen
ISBN 1 84310 743 0

Hitchhiking through Asperger Syndrome
Lise Pyles
Foreword by Tony Attwood
ISBN 1 85302 937 8

Freaks, Geeks and Asperger Syndrome
A User Guide to Adolescence
Luke Jackson
Foreword by Tony Attwood
ISBN 1 84310 098 3

The Development of Autism
A Self-Regulatory Perspective
Thomas L. Whitman
ISBN 1 84310 735 X

To all those who *genuinely cared* for the three of us:

To the memory of
Dobrila and Milivoje Vuletic,
Adrien Pinard, and
Ana and Constantin Mihail

And to
Djordje Sredojevic,
Diane, Marcel, and Cynthia Ferrari,
Silvia and Adrian Mihail, and
Costel and Elena Poterasu

Contents

List of Figures and Tables

Figures

Table

Acknowledgements

We would like to thank many people who helped us in various ways while we were preparing this book.

Teodor would like to thank his parents Silvia and Adrian Mihail, for being patient with him and teaching him to be a good student, positive, polite, respectful, self-confident, and many other things he can't even remember; his grandparents Costel and Elena Poterasu, for caring for him, loving him no matter what he does, and for teaching him so many things, too many to mention; and his friend Kevin (not his real name, but he knows who he is), for being his best friend for six years, for helping him realize how his "funny sounds" are not funny to other people in school, and for a million other things.

Ljiljana would like to thank her husband Djordje Sredojevic, for his love, care, encouragement, and support, as well as for his help with images for this book; her son Petar Sredojevic, for adding variety to her life, including humor and new perspectives on life, and for his help with editing several versions of this book and correcting many misplaced English articles; her sister Milena Djolovic and her aunt Vida Veskovic for their love and support; all the autistic children and their families who taught her about autism – Teodor and his parents, Silvia and Adrian Mihail in particular; Teodor's parents, grandparents and teaching assistant for agreeing to be interviewed, and for reading and commenting on the manuscript; Teodor's friend Kevin (not his real name), for providing his autobiography and Teodor's biography; and her friends and colleagues for their support, encouragement, understanding, and/or reading portions of the manuscript, in particular to Helena and Vlade Jovanovic, Verica and Nenad Milic, Dijana Plut, Joan Moss, Susan London McNab, Freya Kristjanson, Andrew Faiz, Emiko Koyama, Eva Filipova, and Nancy Smart.

Michel would like to thank his parents, family, friends, and students who together have given him the support and strength to see and explore the world in new ways.

Ljiljana and Michel would both like to thank Dr Nancy Link, for her help with the *WISC-III* testing and interpreting, for her critical reading of part of the book, and for her thoughtful comments; and Dr

Joe Ducharme, for his helpful comments on the initial draft of the manuscript.

Special thanks from all three authors go to Jessica Kingsley and her publishing team for their editorial advice and enormous patience with us in bringing this book to fruition.

Note to reader

This book is about its third author, Teodor Mihail, who provided autobiographical material for the book. All interpretations are made by Ljiljana Vuletic and Michel Ferrari, except when specifically noted otherwise. All reviews and connecting narratives in the book are also Ljiljana and Michel's. Wherever possible, we have tried to separate our interpretations from our data or reviews of scholarly evidence. Our personal opinions can be found in the *Commentaries* and *Reflections* sections. However, a lot of raw material has been left uninterpreted —this book would never have been published had we done otherwise.

All names, except for those of the authors, are psuedonyms.

1

A Transfer Boy

A small group of children are chaotically moving around, bragging about video games, trading hockey cards and pushing each other for no reason at all as the group's instructor prepares to begin the community centre's after-school class of "mind games." In the far corner of the room, an eight-year-old boy sits at a small table. He appears to be drawing. One boy from the group of children notices the boy in the corner, approaches him, and asks: "What are you doing?"

"None of your business," he replies, in a firm high-pitched voice, looking at the boy in front of him for only a split-second before continuing.

"Is that a bus ticket?" the standing boy asks, pointing to a small brownish piece of paper covered with lines, numbers and letters.

"NO, it's a bus TRANSfer," the seated boy replies, in the same firm high-pitched voice, without interrupting his activity.

"Why are you copying a bus TRANSfer?" the boy asks, looking at another piece of paper on which the seated boy is writing numbers and making lines like those on the transfer.

"None of your business," the seated boy replies, in the same firm voice, then jerks his head back, away from the boy in front of him, and stays in that position for a moment as if frozen. The other boy raises his eyebrows, pouts his lips, shrugs, turns around and walks towards the group of children at the big table. The seated boy resumes his interrupted activity.

The group instructor is now announcing the beginning of the games session and invites the children to sit around the big table in the middle of the room. The children are now frantically moving around. In a few seconds everyone is seated at a big table, except for the boy in the corner. The group leader invites him to join the rest of his classmates. The boy, still looking at the table in front of him, answers, in a robot-like voice: "I-DON'T-HAVE-TO-play."

"No, you don't have to, but if you WANT TO, you can join us."

"My-mother-said-I-DON'T-HAVE-TO-PLAY."

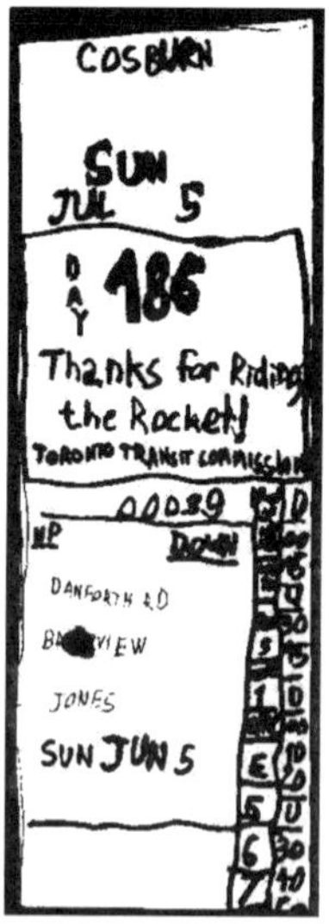

Figure 1.1: The boy's copy of a bus transfer

"No, you don't have to," the group leader replies in a calm and reassuring voice, turns back to the group of children around the big table, and starts to explain the rules of the game they will play. All the while, the boy in the corner continues copying his transfer.

Half an hour later, a girl stands up and moves closer to the boy in the corner. She stands beside him, observes him for a moment and then asks in a soft voice:

"Why don't you want to play with us?"

"I-don't-HAVE-TO-play!" the boy replies, in the same high-pitched mechanical voice as before, still copying, as before.

"Why don't you WANT to play with us?" the girl tries again, standing there for another minute and watching what the boy is doing.

"I-don't-want-to-play!" The boy with the transfers replies, uninterruptedly, in an ever-raising voice.

The girl, still standing there, leaning ever closer to the table, examines the two pieces of paper in front of the boy. The boy, now interrupting his work, yells:

"LEAVE-ME-ALONE!"

Ever since this episode, the group instructor, also the first author of this book, has been trying to understand this physically present, but mentally absent, "transfer boy." She hoped to break through his invisible barrier and gain access to that other world where she felt he existed. This book is written, in part, as a record of this effort.

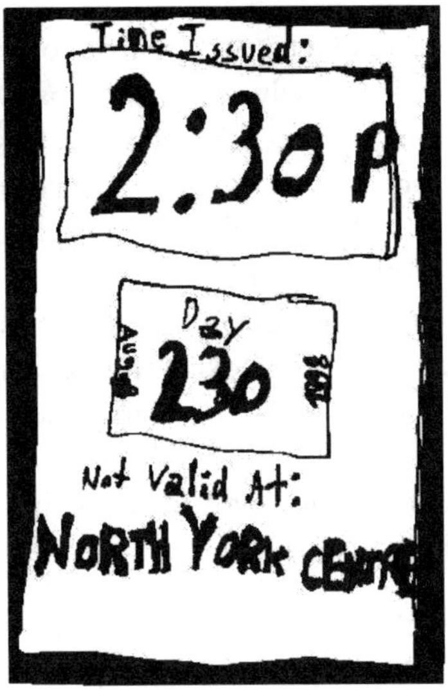

Figure 1.2: The boy's copy of a subway transfer

The transfer boy, Teodor, is not a typical child: he does not seem to be at all interested in what his peers are doing when they joke around and play group games. Instead, he does things his peers would probably find boring—copies letters, numbers, and words from one piece of paper to another. And not just one copy, but many, without anybody asking him, and for a long period of time with the highest level of concentration. Not only does Teodor seem disinterested in what other children are doing, but he actually avoids them—he sits in the corner alone and answers their questions defensively ("I don't have to") or by verbally pushing them away ("None of your business" and "Leave me alone"). But although Teodor is not a typical child, he is also not alone.

In fact, there are many children like Teodor—children who came to scientific and clinical attention some eighty years ago. Clinical descriptions say that such children:

> are occupied by an action, they aim at one goal, they are involved with the things in their activities and although, or perhaps because, they are totally involved, they remain unaffected, unresponding, unmoved by many things that would affect, move, and evoke response from other people in a similar situation. (Bosch 1962/1970, p.52)

The Austrian pediatrician Hans Asperger was among the first to describe them. According to his description of an eight-and-a-half-year-old child, Harro L., "One would never see him join in a game with others. Most of the time, he sat in a corner buried in a book, oblivious to the noise or movement around him" (1944/1991, p.56). "He talked slowly and in a deadpan way without much modulation. He never looked at his interlocutor while talking" (p.52). "His facial expressions were sparse and rigid. With this went a general stiffness and clumsiness" (p.57). He also adds, "The peculiarities of Harro's behavior can all be explained in terms of his contact disturbance, that is, his extremely limited relationship to his environment" (p.56). But, "Although he was aloof from things and people—or perhaps because of this—he had rich experiences and his own independent interests" (p.52). Asperger called Harro and other children like him *autistic.*[1]

In 1926, in what is currently believed to be the first clinical account of such children, Russian neurologist Ewa Ssucharewa spoke of "an autistic attitude":

> All affected children keep themselves apart from their peers, find it hard to adapt to and are never fully themselves among other children. [...] All these children manifest a tendency towards solitude and avoidance of other people from early childhood onwards; they keep themselves apart, avoid communal games and prefer fantastic stories and fairy tales. (Quoted in Wolff 1996, p.129)

Today's scientific literature refers to children like Teodor—who avoid communication and social interaction, have extremely high interest in a few circumscribed topics, or engage in stereotyped behaviors—as "having" autism, Autistic Disorder, autistic spectrum disorder, Pervasive Developmental Disorder (PDD), high-functioning autism, Asperger's Disorder (or syndrome), or nonverbal learning disability.[2]

This book aims to understand Teodor as a person by coordinating the views of him from different perspectives obtained in different contexts and at different times (see Appendix A for details). We will get to know Teodor from the perspectives of his family (his parents and grandparents), his school staff (his teacher and former teaching assistant), his psychiatrist, and from his own perspective. And although each person (unusual or not) is unique, he or she also shares many features with others. As far as we are successful in understanding Teodor, at least some of our insights could be generalized to apply to others like him. Our second aim is to use the multifaceted understanding that we arrive at to find ways to broaden Teodor's world.

2

A Good and Loving Child

The Family Perspective

In this section we get to know twelve-year-old Teodor as his family members see him. We hear the voices of his parents—Sandra and Andrew, both in their early forties—and of his maternal grandparents—Helen, in her late sixties, and Radu, in his early seventies—as they talk with Teodor and about Teodor with the first author of this book, Ljiljana.

"Don't go beyond the yellow line!": The grandmother's perspective

Teodor:	Grandma, could we go to on a trip to Newmarket tomorrow?
Grandma:	Depends how long it will take.
Teodor:	According to my plan we first take the GO bus to Newmarket, then take the Highway 400 GO bus to Yorkdale, then to get home we need to take a subway, bus 165 or 96 to York Mills, then the subway to Finch and the GO bus from Finch to Richmond Hill. So that is going to be approximately five to six hours. Is that OK?
Grandma:	Not quite.
Teodor:	What if it is a four-hour trip?
Grandma:	That is OK.
Teodor:	OK then, I'll change the plan so that the trip is four hours.
Grandma:	OK.

Teodor opens a transit map, inspects it carefully for the bus schedule, writes down some numbers, looks at the map again, then repeats this sequence a few more times; then he looks at the map of another town, inspects it for a few moments, looks at another brochure, and so on. A little later, he comes to his grandma and tells her his new plan, including the bus and train routes they will be taking and their approximate length; he gives his grandma a worried look, and asks her again, "Is that all right with you?" After his grandma confirms, he smiles at her and exclaims happily, "Oh good!"

The next day, on their way to the bus stop, Teodor walks a few steps ahead of his grandma. From time to time, he stops, turns around and asks, "Am I going too fast?", his grandma says no, he slows down to grandma's pace for a while, then walks faster again. After a while he turns around again, sees his grandma a few steps behind and asks her, "Are you all right?" Teodor's grandma answers yes, and they continue to walk at the same pace for a while. This repeats a few more times: Teodor stops, turns around, realizes that his grandma is walking slower and slower, asks her whether or not she is OK, then slows down for a bit, and then accelerates again. As they get closer to the bus stop, Teodor starts looking at his watch from time to time. When they get to where they might see the bus coming, Teodor adds looking in the direction of the bus to his sequence. At the bus stop, Teodor tells his grandma that there is no bus in sight, looks around, finds her a bench in the shade and tells her to sit there. He looks at his watch, and tells his grandma how long they will have to wait. Then he asks her a series of questions: "Are you all right?, Do you need something?, Are you thirsty?, Are you hungry?" After his grandma reassures him that she is OK, he looks again to see if the bus is coming.

When the bus comes, Teodor helps his grandma get on the bus, pays the fare, asks the bus driver for two transfers, and finds two seats. Once they are both sitting, he carefully inspects the new transfers for a few minutes. Then he opens his bag, takes out a metal box he calls his "bank" (Figures 2.1 and 2.2), turns the combination numbers on the lock, opens the box, carefully places the transfers in it, closes the box, locks it, and then puts it back into his bag. He begins to look through the window, and when the bus passes an interesting building, Teodor tells his grandma what it is. When they get to the subway station, Teodor asks his grandma, "Do you wanna go to the bathroom?" and "Do you need anything?" He then tells her that he needs to copy some transit information into his notebook, finds a bench for her nearby and starts to copy. From time to time, he looks back at his grandma and asks, "Are you all right?" or "Are you bored?" When his grandma reassures him that she is OK, he continues his "work." When he is done, he informs his grandma that they will be continuing their trip and asks her, "Do you wanna take the escalator or the stairs?" When they get to the subway platform, Teodor warns his grandma, "Don't go beyond the yellow line!" He also tells her how far they are going. Then he repeats the sequence of finding the bench, checking the time, checking whether the train is coming, and checking whether his grandma is OK a few more times with some variations before they return home.

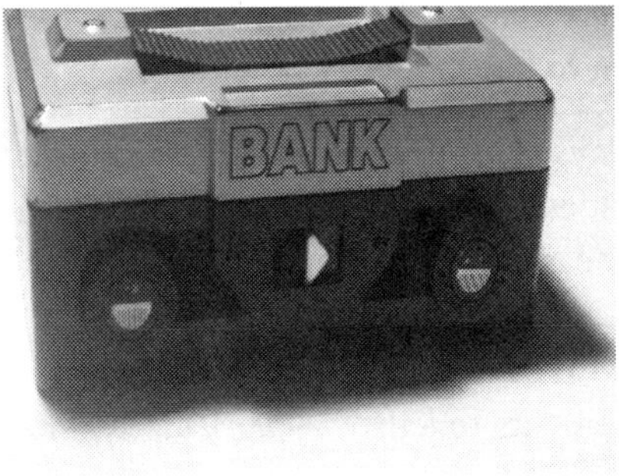

Figure 2.1: Teodor's "bank" from the outside

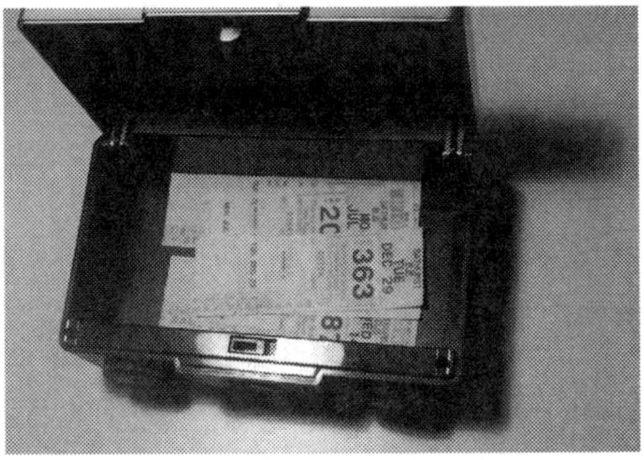

Figure 2.2: The inside of Teodor's "bank"

When they get back, Teodor happily informs the family at home that the trip was great, and tells them many details about the buses and trains they took, the transfers they got, and information he copied into his notebook. Finally, Teodor goes to his room, takes the notebook and the "bank" out of his bag, takes the transfers from the "bank" and spends the next few hours studying the transfers and the new information, "making a good copy" of the new information in another notebook, and putting everything in its proper place.

Teodor's grandmother, Helen, has cared for Teodor for almost his whole life. She was the first to notice something unusual about Teodor when he was about four years old. Helen was born and lived most of her life in Romania. She came to Canada when Teodor was nine years old. Since she does not speak English, Teodor's mother (her daughter) served as interpreter during the interview with Ljiljana. (This is why third-person pronouns—"she" and "her"—appear in her interview statements instead of first-person pronouns—"I" and "me.")

During the interview, Helen often says that she loves Teodor very much and that he is "her soul." She feels that Teodor loves her too:

> Teodor very often says that he doesn't want to get far [away] from [his grandmother]—never. He doesn't imagine her leaving him—never. When she is upset and she is telling him that she is upset and she is gonna leave and she is gonna go back to Romania—so she is gonna be more quiet and everything[3]—he always just do[es] whatever she asks him—immediately.

She adds:

> He is a very good child. He has a very warm soul. He is a little bit selfish. And he doesn't have confidence in all the people—the people around, including the kids, his friends. He gets [finds making] friends very hard. He thinks that people around want to hurt him. Like the kids in school or somebody else—like they would want to hurt him somehow.

Helen also said that usually before he plays with children, she first needs to reassure him that, "This is a good child, he doesn't want to hurt you—it's no harm for you." After that, she added, "he can get easily friends, but he has to pass this barrier of not trusting people and seeing the people around like enemies."

Teodor is very friendly and caring towards his grandmother: "He always goes to her, and they have their own lovely moments together"—particularly when they go on trips together:

> When they are going together on the TTC,[4] he is really taking care of her—he is always asking her, Are you all right? Am I going too fast? Do you wanna to go to the bathroom? Do you wanna take the escalator? Do you wanna take the stairs? Do you need something? Are you thirsty? Are you hungry? [...] He is really, really taking care of her. [...] He is very, very careful when he is with her and he is taking care of her really well. And she likes that. He explains to her where did they go, what it is there and all the things.

However, there are times when Teodor is "naughty." "Like when he answers back or when sometimes she is asking him to do something, he would say—sometimes, 'I'm gonna do it later' or 'Ah, you are always bothering me when I am busy'—and things like that." Teodor's grandmother would also like Teodor to be less "messy." However, she adds, smiling, that even though she does not always like his behavior, she always likes to look at him since he is a very handsome boy.

"Don't forget to make the cross sign!": The grandfather's perspective

Teodor and his grandfather are playing the board game "Dinosaur."

Teodor: Dinosaur! [In a high-pitched voice.]

Grandpa: Ah, ah—it's not nice, it's not nice. [In a deep and caring voice, perhaps thinking that Teodor was making reference to him.]

Teodor: Ah, ah—it's not nice, it's not nice. [In the same bass voice as his grandpa, and laughing right after he said it.]

Grandpa: Not nice. [In a deep and stern voice.]

Teodor: It's SO funny how you said it, "Ah, ah—it's not nice, it's not nice." [Continues to laugh for several more seconds.] SO funny. [He makes his move and they continue the game.]

[Before the game ends, Teodor repeats a few more times]

Teodor: Dinosaur! [In a high-pitched voice.] Ah, ah—it's not nice, it's not nice. [In a deep voice; laughs for several seconds.] It's SO funny.

Teodor's grandfather, Radu, is caring and an avid advocate of discipline. He likes to play chess and card games with Teodor. He, too, spent most of his life in Romania and came to Canada when Teodor was nine years old. And since he also does not speak English, Teodor's mother (his daughter) interpreted the interview with Ljiljana.

Radu gives the following description of Teodor:

> Teodor is a very nice grandson and—from the moment he came here three years ago—Teodor's behavior improved a lot towards him. So he thinks that he [Teodor] is a good boy and he is somewhat disciplined... When he said 'disciplined' he actually referred to the fact that he [Teodor] has respect towards the older people.

Radu believes that Teodor is "improving" in other areas as well. He said:

> Teodor is improving. So his path is on the improving side on day-to-day life and school life... Before he was very nervous, very angry all the time—now he is not so much any more.

However, he feels that there are still some areas in which his grandson could improve, particularly in his [Teodor's] interaction and communication with his peers. From his perspective, "Teodor doesn't have the cooperation with the kids at his age." In addition, he said:

> He is too childish for his age... When he just talks to the kids—and the TTC—he emphasizes too much on this TTC, not like kids at his age that would have different other interests.

When asked to share some special moments he had with his grandson, he remembered the pleasure Teodor's behavior gave him on their trips when Teodor was four or five years old:

> This happened in Romania. And he [Radu] cannot forget this—when they were in the transit in Romania—the same as TTC here—and when somebody old—that [was] in the bus—Teodor will always just get up and offer that [his] seat to that person. And another thing is that whenever he passes a church he would make the sign—the cross [Romanian custom among older people]—and sometimes when my father didn't see the

church or something, he would point it to my father, like, "Here is the church, don't forget to make the cross sign."

"If he were a millionaire, he would want a bus": The mother's perspective

> I remember the first time—I think Teodor was three—when we first took him with a train... I think that for the first one hour—I would say one hour—he wouldn't even move. I had to feel that [whether] he was breathing or not because he was petrified—not like fear petrified, but just petrified. I wouldn't even know if he liked it or not because he wouldn't say a word, he wouldn't move—not even his eyes... I will never forget this, and I really analyzed it but I never came to a conclusion about it. I would say it was pleasure but, like, it was the first thing for him and he was really, like—I never expected this kind of thing... Because all the things were happening, like the conductor will come to see the tickets and stuff, and you know, that would just distract him—it won't—like, it just didn't happen—he didn't move, he didn't—I was afraid that he didn't even breathe. [smiles] This was *the* thing... He was just like that [tensing her body and opening her eyes, as if in a state of maximum alertness]. I would say it was a kind of ecstasy kind of thing—I wouldn't know that. He wasn't scared—that's for sure. He wasn't scared because the kids at this age would cry or stuff like that—he won't. But I would say it was ecstasy, but I don't know.

Teodor's mother, Sandra, is an engineer, energetic, ambitious, and self-confident. She came to Canada when Teodor was five years old and is optimistic and determined to do whatever it takes to help Teodor live a happy and productive life. She describes him in the following way:

> Teodor is a very loving child—a very loving child and I really appreciate that. His behavior is good in regard to rules, so I won't have a problem with him just having to be against the rules. He would listen to the rules... Like, let's say he won't be, like, nasty with the people on the bus, or he won't go on the bus thinking not to pay, or he would cross the street properly, things like this.

However, Teodor has difficulties interacting with other children:

> He is a little bit not comfortable with, like, a big group of people. When he is with other kids he would try to impose his way of playing, and if they don't want to play his game he's not very respective of their way of playing. So he would try to do something else without bothering other people. He won't do anything to bother other kids, but he would do his own

> stuff—drawing or looking at his schedules and stuff like that. And so his interaction with kids is not so good. He is very comfortable with kids smaller then he is, and he would play nicely with them, and they'd like him very much, probably because he is big and they like that, and probably because he likes to fool around, like the small kids do, so they appreciate that.

Also, Sandra has noticed that Teodor "likes playing with girls" and has recently "started looking at the girls"—in a romantic way. For example, he would make new kinds of comments about girls, such as, "I really like this girl. She looks so nice. She is so pretty."

Even though, typically, Teodor's interactions with children are not very good, in some situations he is "very understanding towards other people—other people's problems." For example, if a friend is hurt, he will try to help: "He would come home, get the band-aid, go there, take care, and just try to help."

With regard to behavior in school, Teodor follows the rules of proper school conduct:

> I don't have problems with Teodor in school because, as I say, he is very good with the rules, and if the teacher said, "You're not allowed to do that," he won't do that. So I don't have problems with the teachers calling me saying that Teodor did this or this and stuff like that.

With regard to academic achievement, Teodor is a "B- kind of student:"

> He is doing math because we are engineers and he knows that math is important because we reinforce that so many times, but not that he likes it. Science—he would do it as a homework kind of thing, but he won't be very interested in that. Reading is—for him reading is a tool to understand his schedules and his TTC stuff and his flight stuff—it's not reading as in literature or other things. He would be—reading is a tool as much as computer is a tool. He won't be interested in knowing how the programs are working or why […] that [is]. He would use the computer the way he uses the pen and the paper. So in school he's okay. Lately he doesn't have the assistant and he is doing much, much better independently, and I really appreciate that.

When it comes to homework, Teodor is very keen on having his homework done:

> He would do his homework regularly and he would ask for help if he doesn't know how to do it, and he cannot understand the concept of […] going to school without the homework done. So he would insist—let's say it's 11 o'clock—I say, "It's time to go to bed right now, you cannot function properly, don't do this homework"—I have to write a note for the teacher

> because he won't go to school without his homework done. That's another rule, and he would follow it—to the end.

However, Teodor is very dependent on parental help for his homework. Sandra feels that, without help, he "would be lost because he won't be able to prioritize things; he won't know what's more important, and not knowing that he would try to do everything but not be able to do it. And that would just build up to a really big frustration." She explained that when she, last semester, tried to "minimize" her help Teodor's "marks went a little bit down." She also added, "But I wanted to experience what's happening when I'm giving him minimal supervision," which she estimated to be around "three hours per week" (for the subjects from her domain of responsibility: social studies, and language arts—her husband is responsible for Teodor's other main academic areas, math and science).

Sandra says that other than having to do homework together, "I don't have major problems with Teodor; I don't have big problems with Teodor—I have normal, regular issues like all the parents have." And she provides the following example of a regular issue:

> He's messy. So I have to say it all over again, "Did you do that and did you do that?" and stuff like that. Lately he got used to making his own bed and cleaning his own room just because he's in the caretaker crew in school, and he got a little bit changed since he started there and he's trying to clean his room better lately. But I would think this is normal at this age and I would think that not paying attention at this is not a big issue.

But there is one thing that Teodor does that really annoys Sandra: Teodor has a habit of making "silly noises" (i.e., imitating sounds made by other people, animals or machines)—a bad habit she hopes he will soon "outgrow."

Other than that, Teodor does fine at home: he is "very polite," he "really loves his family," and in general is "really well related to the family." Sandra feels that this is one of the similarities between her son and herself at his age. "I was considerate towards my family and so is he." However, she also found some differences between them:

> If I compare him with me, like—I was very much into reading and watching movies, and thinking about myself in a, like, a different world that I would see in those books, and try to put myself in those situations and exploring a lot with my mind—what's going to happen if, how would I be if, and stuff like that—while he's not at all interested in that. He lives in reality and he won't think about him living in poverty in Mexico[5]—he would never ever think about this. Or how would he be if he would live in Robin Hood's time—he would never think about that.

The young Sandra and her son were also very different in their social needs:

> I was very much interested in being in a group while he's not. I wanted very much to have friends; well, this is not his main priority. If he has friends—that's fine, if he doesn't—that's fine. He's not looking for friends while I was. And he won't like being in a group and doing whatever everybody would do—he would want to do his stuff. And he doesn't want to be popular. He doesn't want to be dressed in certain clothes. This is not one of his problems.

In reconstructing her view of the world at Teodor's age, and comparing it to his, Sandra finds that they share a similar optimistic tone, although founded on different grounds:

> I thought that the world is great and I did have this optimism that everything is possible and I can do whatever I want if I want to do that. Like, for Teodor, I don't even think that he has, like, a global kind of view about this, but for him too, the world didn't hurt him yet, so he thinks about—this is what I think is—that he thinks that the world is a place he likes to be in, and I don't think that he placed himself in the world yet. I don't think that he has this kind of capacity of picturing him. But I think he feels good, and the world for him is good.

In the future, Sandra pictures Teodor doing something involving buses and trains. She said, "I mostly see Teodor doing kind of a scheduling for TTC or for railway if there is such a thing." However, while trying to imagine Teodor in the future, she recalls situations in which Teodor cares about other people, and from this perspective, she believes that Teodor could have a career working with others:

> I really imagine Teodor working with people that need help. I would say like a social work kind of thing, like a person or—not like a psychologist—more like working with people that have the same difficulties as he has... I would see Teodor interacting with this kind of people the way he interacts with small kids right now. And because he's very loving and considerate I would think he would make a very good—like a big brother kind of thing. Like, you know, they have those programs called Big Brother [*Big Brothers, Big Sisters,* the largest youth one-to-one mentoring organization in the US] when the people that have problems would need somebody else to spend some time with them or something like that. So I would see Teodor working with people with special needs.

Finally, Sandra believes that if her son were a millionaire, "he would want a bus."

"I was the same": The father's perspective

> [When I was twelve] I was interested in what Teodor is interested [in] now—with some exceptions. He's very good in Lego—now he went up one level building all these planes and assembly and gluing and painting—his planes, cars, ships—whatever... I was the same. I was building this kind of toy by myself, the same model kits.

Teodor's father, Andrew, an engineer, is energetic, self-confident and easy-going. He is a strong opponent of punitive disciplinary methods and says this about Teodor:

> He is somehow different than the other children because he likes to live how he likes, and if this kind of living is in contradiction with what all the other children are doing, he's trying to go on his way.

In comparing himself to Teodor when he was his age, Andrew said:

> I think Teodor is at the bottom [of the group of peers]; he's not rejected but has trouble of being part of the group. Sometimes being targeted, but it's still part of the group—I mean he's not an outsider, or probably somewhere in there... I didn't have problems having friends... When I was a kid I was, let's say—not a leader, but under—the next—close, but not the leader—never the leader... I was under—immediately under—which is a difference if I compare with Teodor.

Andrew believes that part of Teodor's difficulty in finding his place in a group of peers stems from his lack of understanding of what friendship is:

> He doesn't understand exactly the relations with a friend. I mean he's extremely selfish. He uses a friend only to please himself without thinking that it should be the other way around the same. I mean he is sometimes pretty cruel with his friends... He's using a friend like a toy—something he needs and he likes, but if the other—if his friend will behave absolutely the same—they cannot be friends.

Andrew also emphasizes an imbalance in Teodor's physical development which seems to be a few years ahead and his mental development which seems to be a few years behind:

> He is like a sixteen-year-old boy. He's one head and a half taller than all these children from his class. And in his class he's okay, but when he's outside...he looks like [a sixteen-year-old]; [they] believe that he's one of them but his brain is not sixteen years old—he's like a twelve-year-old with a sixteen-year-old body, and probably ten-year-old's brain... When

> he's outside of the class—in school or on the street or everywhere—everybody judges him like [a] sixteen-year-old—and he's not—he's not even twelve.

However, Andrew feels that Teodor includes the family in his world, and that within the family he is "getting along *better* than outside." This is because the family members tolerate all Teodor's behavior, which is not the case outside the family. Here is Andrew's perception of the "game" in which Teodor imitated his grandfather's voice:

> He picks a proposition—or somebody says something—and starts repeating all over again. I mean he makes a game and then—for him it's funny—let's say in a dialog—he picks two—a statement and an answer, and then he make this like a game, and he's repeating it for three-four months—he doesn't forget that thing... [For example,] he said, "Dinosaur" to somebody—to his grandfather—and his grandfather said, "Ah, ah—it's not nice, it's not nice." ... And he likes this, and now he plays the game.

Even though Teodor's father does not like these "games," he does not try to stop Teodor from playing them:

> If you say, "You cannot play this anymore. Stop. Stop doing it," he will react extremely hard, I know. And I think it's better to play just a little bit, let's say, one week—two weeks and then he will forget. Otherwise, it will take more and if he cannot say these, he will concentrate to find something else. And then if you want to find something else, you won't find one, maybe you'll find two or three. And you'll say, "Don't do this—don't say this," and they will say three things instead of one. So you better let it with that one and he will forget in time, and maybe it will be less and less things to repeat.

Andrew said that Teodor was very willing to please his parents, but was unresponsive to punishment. Thus when Teodor was punished for engaging in a particular activity, he would nevertheless continue with that activity. This is "exactly opposite" to how Andrew reacted in the same situation when he was Teodor's age. He says, "I was pretty sensitive to punishment; I mean, when I was ten—twelve, I didn't like to go to school. So after I [got] punished my grades went up a lot." To the contrary,

> [Teodor] is extremely sensitive to reward. If you reward him, you can do anything you want. I mean—let's say his hobby with trips—I promise him that—this is more than he can imagine—a trip to Montreal by train—and I told him that he will get this reward if two thirds of his tests will be A and B, and just one third C... He's so excited and if he won't do it, that means this is his level—I mean, he cannot do any better. But he's so focused on

> this and—I mean when we have—I teach him math and science and when he has a test, if he knows that there is a reward—and always there is a reward if he take an A or B—he comes to me and says "Let's repeat one more time to be sure that I know everything and tomorrow I get A." This is a wonderful tool.

In school, Teodor's father believes that Teodor is "somewhere in the middle—not between the brightest but not the last one." He also believes that Teodor has a "very emotional approach to a learning process"—a characteristic they share; for example, he refuses to learn things he dislikes. Thus, Teodor "refuse[s] to pay attention" to stories and to anything "related to social skills." "If you read a book to him, you can see that he's thinking about something else." Andrew said that he too refused to learn things that he didn't like and that, like Teodor, he did not like languages. On the other hand, "It's easy to teach [him] math [and] science," since he is "focusing and learning very fast." He believes that Teodor is, in fact, very interested in these two subjects.

When Andrew imagines Teodor in the future, he cannot picture Teodor having a job in which he would have to "manage people." On the other hand, he can easily imagine Teodor having a variety of jobs related to science:

> Definitely [I cannot see Teodor] in a job that will require social skills, like teacher or something that have to work or manage people. I can see him working in an environment where his job is related more to selfwork—like, a computer scientist—writing programs for a computer—all kind of activities, I think, related to science. I cannot imagine him like a lawyer. Or, if he cannot go to university, let's say he got some business administration college or something like this—I don't think he will be good in this, or [if] he can do it. Just in jobs related more with working in small teams—by himself—not exposed to big groups or something like that. Or if [he] will work—I cannot see him going up in management or something like that because I don't think he can—but there are lot of—depend[ing] on his ability to learn—which—if, let's say, won't improve—which is hard to believe—but let's say will not improve—and will be in the middle—with this middle, there are lot of jobs that he can take and have a reasonable career.

When searching for unforgettable moments with Teodor, his father remembered their trips:

> Probably—will be in my memory—our trips with trains and buses together. I didn't enjoy too much but he enjoys [them] a lot and that's something different—this will remain probably in my mind. He is so happy—his face is like a sun.

Commentary: The family's portrait of Teodor

Teodor enjoys a prominent place in his family—he is unconditionally loved by all its members; whenever possible, his wishes are fulfilled and his learning efforts are supported. Looking more closely at family members' accounts of Teodor, we find more similarities than differences. They most often agree in their general characterizations of Teodor but disagree on specifics, such as how to interpret Teodor's behavior.

All family members agreed that Teodor is, first and foremost, a good and loving child. Thus, in describing Teodor, his family members used words such as good, nice, loving, caring, disciplined, and polite. They also said that he has a "warm soul," "good intentions," and "respect towards older people," and that he "really loves his family." The fact that he is also sometimes "naughty" did not influence the family's general perception of Teodor as a good child.

All family members agree that Teodor has some difficulties interacting and communicating with other children. However, they disagree about how serious these difficulties are and what causes them. Teodor's mother believes that Teodor's main difficulty is his "not [being] comfortable with a big group of people," which, from her perspective, is just a matter of priorities: Teodor just happens to have other priorities—"his TTC stuff." Teodor's grandmother sees Teodor's interaction difficulties as stemming from lack of confidence in other people, especially other children. His grandfather believes that Teodor's lack of common interests with his peers and his "childish" preoccupation with the TTC are to blame for these difficulties. Likewise, Teodor's father believes that Teodor's most serious difficulty is "being part of the group"; Teodor's father identifies three potential reasons for this difficulty. First, Teodor refuses to accept other children's ways of playing. Second, he does not understand friendship and "uses a friend like a toy," without considering the friend's needs and wishes. However, Teodor's father also thinks that other children's perceptions of Teodor as a boy older than his real age contribute to his son's difficulties in social interaction.

All family members also agree that the TTC has a special place in Teodor's life, although there are some differences of opinion about how special it is and whether this focus is good or bad (or neither). Teodor's mother assigns it the most important place in Teodor's life, referring to it as Teodor's "priority," and calling it simply "Teodor's stuff." She considered Teodor very different from herself at his age; while she wanted to be part of a group of children, "he would want to do his stuff." Her comment that if Teodor were a millionaire "he would want a bus" is a good illustration of how important she thinks the TTC interest is to Teodor. She interpreted Teodor's first train trip experience as a "kind of ecstasy kind of thing," and when asked to imagine Teodor in the future, her first thought was of Teodor "scheduling for TTC or for [a] railway." Teodor's grandfather provides the second most explicit position on Teodor's interest in the TTC. He says that Teodor "emphasizes too much on this TTC." Although Teodor's father also remembered their bus and train trips as the most unforgettable moments with his son, because on these trips Teodor is "so happy—his face is like a sun," he did not talk much about them, nor did he think that this "hobby" will necessarily find a place in Teodor's career. However, by using it as a tool to motivate Teodor to do schoolwork, he implicitly acknowledges the great importance of the TTC in Teodor's life. He knows that when he promises Teodor a bus or train trip as a reward for good marks, Teodor will do his best. Finally, even though Teodor's grandmother did not talk specifically about Teodor's interest in the TTC, she, too, chose to share memories from trips with Teodor as the most unforgettable moments they spent together.

As to whether Teodor's TTC interest is good or bad (or neither), Teodor's grandfather seems to be the only member of the family who is concerned about it. He sees it as something very "childish," which somehow prevents him from having other interests. In his view, Teodor would be much better off if he had interests more similar to those of his peers. Teodor's father, on the other hand, looks at his son's interest in the TTC as a "wonderful tool" for motivating him, but not as having a value in itself. For Teodor's mother, on the other hand, not only does her son's interest in the TTC have a value in itself, but she believes that it might become his future career. Finally, Teodor's grandmother has never refused to accompany Teodor on his trips, so she probably perceives Teodor's TTC interest as unproblematic.

All in all, regardless of their different views on the role and value of Teodor's TTC interests, by choosing to share their experiences from their trips with Teodor (rather than "home events"), all family members acknowledged that Teodor's TTC interest has a prominent place in their family life. It not only occupies most of Teodor's time, but also impacts on the life of his whole family.

Neither of Teodor's parents approves of the way Teodor has fun imitating sounds, and they both spoke about their struggle to find the best way to help Teodor "outgrow it." While Teodor's father believes that ignoring this kind of play is the best approach, Teodor's mother uses canceling TTC trips or taking away Teodor's favorite desserts and sweets if he does not stop when reminded once. Teodor's grandfather's reaction to Teodor's imitation of his voice shows that he too does not approve of this kind of "having fun," but his own gentle way of dealing with it is to tell Teodor that it is "not nice."

Teodor is an average student overall, and above average in mathematics and science. However, Teodor's parents have different explanations for Teodor's relatively better success in these two subjects. Seeing that it is easier to teach Teodor mathematics and science than other subjects, Teodor's father concludes that Teodor is intrinsically motivated to learn these subjects; however, Teodor's mother believes that Teodor's motivation is extrinsic. She says that both she and her husband put a special emphasis on math and science, including hours of extra help, and that that help is apparent in Teodor's relatively better marks in these subjects.[6]

Teodor's parents imagine the future Teodor in quite different working environments. While Teodor's father strongly believes that Teodor could do well in a variety of science-related jobs, Teodor's mother is almost certain that Teodor will have a job related to the TTC. In addition, while Teodor's father—drawing on Teodor's difficulties in interacting with his peers—firmly believes that Teodor could not work in a job that requires working with other people, his mother—drawing on Teodor's sensitivity to other people's problems—believes that Teodor could do well on exactly this kind of a job, provided the people need some kind of help.

This family account gives us a picture of Teodor at home. But it is also important to consider Teodor in other contexts. Like most children, Teodor spends most of his time at school.

3

A Good and Well-Behaved Student

The School Perspective

I made a schedule. (I am pretending to be a driver, and I drive the bus. The bus company is "SRT" (School Region Transit)). Depart class for playground (at recess) at 10:15 (when recess starts) and arrive playground at 10:20. Depart playground for class at 10:40, when bell rings. After staying in class a long time (until I'm done eating my lunch), I leave to go wash desks. The schedule says that the bus operates to room # 102 (before I turn back). After staying in class until the day is over, I depart for the school bus loop. Then, the bus becomes out of service. A driver is waiting to take it to the garage. If I'm behind schedule because the teacher kept us in class for 5–10 minutes, I pretend to call that driver so he doesn't get worried. The schedule also has "operating days" (if Tuesday I have band, the schedule says that Tuesday, the bus terminates in the music room (doesn't operate to room # 102, because I don't wash desks that day). If I observe that the bus is behind/ahead of schedule almost every day, I make schedule changes.

Teodor's account of how he spends his recess

Teodor currently attends grade seven regular class and has an Individual Education Plan (IEP) for English. For the last three years, Teodor had a teaching assistant (TA). Last year, he "shared" his teaching assistant with a few other children in his class. This year, school staff concluded that Teodor does not need any extra help, so he will not have a teaching assistant next year.

"His world revolves around transportation": The teaching assistant's perspective

Teodor had the same teaching assistant for three years. This interview was conducted at the end of the third year when Teodor was twelve:

> His world revolves around transportation—I mean trains—I don't think he sees the whole picture beyond—what's out there. And, like, the kids right now—the twelve-year-old—they're, like, looking, you know, they're—girlfriends and boyfriends and the high school—I don't think Teodor is there yet, you know. I don't see him at that point yet, so his world is very isolated—in his world of his transfers, his world that he's created.

The teaching assistant also noticed some other idiosyncrasies:

> He has some mannerisms that are very different than some of the other kids. He'll make outbursts or he'll repeat sometimes what we say. Like, for example, I'll say, "Guys, sit down," and all of a sudden you hear him say, "Guys, sit down!" out of the blue. And also he has this fantasy—not a fantasy but his savings box (Figures 3.1 and 3.2) on his desk which continues to grow every year, but that's his—and his signs, he has signs and pictures and transfers, which is very different from the other twelve-year-old kids that he's with in the class.

With regard to Teodor's relationship with his peers, his teaching assistant said:

> At first I was very worried about his social interaction with other kids, but that has improved greatly since the first time I worked with him three years ago. He has so many friends in the classroom; he participates in everything in class. He is a typical, I think, a typical twelve-year-old boy... He is involved in everything outside—this year he has been involved in a program at our school—he's helping the custodian clean—it's a whole group of people doing all that. And so he's involved in a group of peers—working with peers cleaning the school—typical—I would say typical twelve-year-old boy.

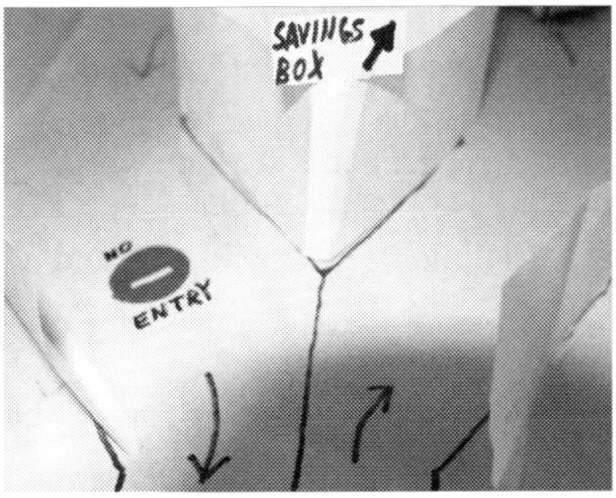

Figure 3.1: Teodor's savings box

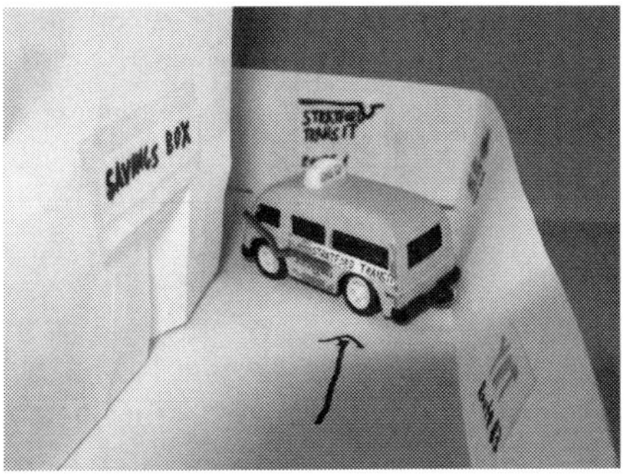

Figure 3.2: Another look at Teodor's savings box

With regard to schoolwork, Teodor "is very independent," "very strong in his science and math," "but languages—that's the weak point for him."

The teaching assistant also noticed that Teodor likes to "make things" and since he also "loves the subway and the trains and the buses" he believes that in the future Teodor will have a career related two these two interests. He said:

> I think I see him almost like an engineer—yeah—of constructing bridges or—he's always making things, he's always building. I think—and with his science and math strength, I mean, I also said that the other day because we were just discussing it because when they leave, you always go, "I wonder what they're going to be in ten years—twenty years from now?"—and I said, "He's going to be building trains or building new subway lines or whatever, or he's going to be an engineer of some sort—building bridges or something." That's how I totally see him.

"In a few instances achieved beyond the standard": The teacher's perspective

No interview with the teacher was conducted due to a scheduling conflict, so her perspective on Teodor is gleaned from her formal assessment of him on his last report card, given at the end of grade six (when he was twelve years old). Here it is in essence:

> ***English:*** Teodor is currently working on a grade level with a few modifications in his reading and writing program...[7] Modifications of additional time, oral discussion and compact lessons. Throughout this term, Teodor's strength in language has been in writing. He has produced work that is well organized and clearly written. Although he includes some good descriptions, he needs to add greater detail... Teodor's written responses demonstrate his increased ability to predict, make judgments and draw conclusions about written works, but lack the details necessary to demonstrate depth of understanding. He continues to respond to written works with concrete understanding, but has difficulty following a text if it is read aloud. (Grades: B-, for all three areas—reading, writing, and oral and visual communication.)
>
> ***French:***[8] Teodor has a good understanding of the vocabulary and structures studied... Written work is completed carefully. Continued active participation is encouraged. (Grades: B+ for oral communication and writing; and B for reading.)
>
> ***Mathematics:*** Teodor has a fair understanding of concepts taught this term. He has not demonstrated consistent ability to explain mathematical processes and strategies using numbers, words and pictures; however, problem

solving is an area in which some growth has been observed over the year. Patterns are sometimes identified but explanations tend to be incomplete. Daily work, homework and journal notes have been good, showing some depth and application of knowledge. The third term math assignments [sic] was completed, demonstrating comprehension of some concepts, but lacking complete explanations. Teodor will benefit from review of grade 6 math concepts over the summer, in preparation for grade 7. I am proud of Teodor's hard work and positive attitude this year. His progress has been admirable. (Grades: B- for geometry and spatial sense; C+ for number sense and numeration; C for measurement and C- for patterning and algebra, and data management and probability.)

Science and technology: Teodor demonstrated good understanding of the basic concepts of the two units studied this term—Motion and Diversity of Living Things. Concepts were related to the real world and communicated with clarity by using appropriate terminology and inquiry skills such as asking questions, planning investigations, recording observations and reaching conclusions. Well done! (Grade: B)

Social studies: At this time Teodor is clearly able to identify ways in which the environment molded Canadian Aboriginal cultures. He is able to describe the impact of early explorers... Teodor would benefit from reading relevant articles in the newspaper to help him maintain his understanding of these issues. (Grade: B)

Health and physical education: Teodor participated with enthusiasm in all activities this term. He attempted all nine events on our track and field days and produced admirable results. In low organization sports, a committed and concerted effort was demonstrated. (Grade: B)

The arts:

Music: Teodor would benefit from being more forthcoming in his response to music... Test results indicate a need for focus and greater effort. (Grade: D-)
Visual arts: This term Teodor has demonstrated careful planning of his work. He made sketches and showed an awareness of the elements and principles of design studied. Teodor chose his colour schemes carefully, and used space effectively. (Grade: B)
Drama and dance: Teodor has difficulty focusing and demonstrating some basic fundamentals of dance this term, including 3-point turns, barrel jumps, box step... Teodor struggled to express himself through interpretation of music. (Grade: C-)

Learning skills: Excellent—for homework completion; Good—for independent work, initiative, use of information, cooperation with others, class participation, and goal setting to improve work; Satisfactory—for conflict resolution, and problem solving.[9]

Strengths/weaknesses/next steps: Teodor has a good year and has seen his efforts produce positive results. He has strived to meet expectations and in a few instances achieved beyond the standard. Teodor has learned how a level-3 response looks and he is learning to answer questions appropriately in this manner. Problem solving has evolved and he used peer and teacher feedback to improve his work. With intensive support, Teodor is becoming a more independent learner. Keep up the great work and good luck in Grade 7.[10]

Commentary

According to school staff, in many ways Teodor is a typical boy for his age and an average student. He is involved in all school activities, both inside and outside the classroom. His interactions with other children are good and he has friends. He participates in class, works independently and completes his homework. He uses peer and teacher feedback to help him set goals and improve his work. According to his teacher, Teodor has some weaknesses in conflict resolution and problem solving; however, this area has been evaluated as at level two (out of four), "satisfactory," and not at the lowest level, "needs improvement."

According to his report card, Teodor's academic performance is relatively consistent and at grade level—even in English for which he has a modified program. However, it should be noted that the teacher's and the teaching assistant's perspectives differ with regard to Teodor's academic strengths. From the teacher's perspective, Teodor's relative strength is in French language, oral communication, and writing (Grade B+), followed by science and technology, social studies, health and physical education and visual arts (Grade B). Teodor's performance in math was evaluated to be on a level C; his lowest grade was in music (Grade D-).

By contrast, from the teaching assistant's perspective, Teodor's strengths are in math and science, and his weakness is in languages. According to him, Teodor is also somewhat unusual in that he has a strong interest in transportation and likes to repeat other people's speech out of context. Still, he finds Teodor's interest in transportation constructive and believes that it will determine Teodor's career path, which he predicts will be in engineering related to trains, subways or bridges.

Reflections

Since the family's perspective on Teodor as a student is based partly on Teodor's report cards and conversations with the teacher and the teaching assistant, it is no surprise that both perspectives yield a very similar portrait. Everybody agrees that Teodor is an average student. Curiously, disagreements are not *between* the family and the school perspectives, rather they are *within* each of these perspectives. Teodor's father and his teaching assistant agree that Teodor's strengths are in math and science, while Teodor's mother and teacher disagree. One way to explain this difference is by looking at who provides Teodor with specific help in these subjects. Teodor's father, who helps Teodor with math and science homework, finds that it is easier for Teodor to learn math and science than other subjects because these subjects matter more to him. Likewise, because Teodor is well prepared in them, he needs less help from the teaching assistant. But both Teodor's mother and his teacher believe that despite getting good marks on assignments that require using mathematical procedures (like division), Teodor's understanding of mathematical concepts remains weak.

Interestingly, family and school perspectives differ regarding Teodor's independent working skills. Both the teacher and the teaching assistant maintain that Teodor's independent working skills are "good," but Teodor's mother feels that Teodor needs specific help setting priorities, at least when it comes to homework. One way to explain this difference is by the different organizational demands of schoolwork and homework. Perhaps Teodor can organize himself within a single class, but not with homework involving different subjects with different due dates.

As for Teodor's social interaction skills, both parents find that Teodor has difficulties in interacting with his peers, whereas the teaching assistant finds Teodor's interaction with his schoolmates adequate both inside and outside the classroom. The teaching assistant's view is partly collaborated by the teacher's evaluation of Teodor's cooperation skills in class; however, the teacher's evaluation of Teodor's conflict resolution skills as merely "satisfactory" partly supports the parental view that Teodor has difficulties in this area. We explain this difference between family and school perspective as follows: the school staff may look at "social interaction" as a dichotomous category (i.e., a child who creates disciplinary problems vs. a child who does not), whereas parents consider the quality of peer interaction. Since Teodor does not create disciplinary problems, the school finds he has no difficulties in this area, but he may still have difficulties interacting with his peers when the quality of interaction is taken into account. Even a superficial look at Figure 3.3 (p.39, in which Teodor lists the activities he engages in during recess) as well as a superficial reading of the introductory story to this chapter clearly shows that Teodor is not in a position to create disciplinary problems because he is not interacting with the children at all—instead he is playing his solitary "games" or engaging in other activities such as drawing, having fun with saying funny things in his head, and occasionally talking to the teacher.

We believe that social competences are as important as academic ones and that social skills are the school's responsibility. We believe that to take part in culture at large, Teodor needs to take part in school culture. His "voluntary" isolation (withdrawal) should be an important problem for school staff, who should help Teodor become more social. We do not think that Teodor's solitary bus-play is appropriate for school recess, because it does not give Teodor the same experience of the playground-world of chase, pretend, chatter, shared joy and excitement, conflict and friendship as it does for other children. If a twelve-year-old boy with his own agenda is left to himself—and to his own agenda—how will he ever be able to take part in any agendas other than his own? And sooner or later he will have to. How will he know what to do—and what not to do, what to say—and what not to say, if he does not start participating *now*? Consider the case of William James Sidis, an extremely gifted person who grew up outside his peer culture and who—as an adult—wrote a book about streetcar transfers—his life-long hobby—that interested no one but him (Winner 1996).[11] We want to make sure that Teodor will use his current interests, or ones he might develop in the future, to create products useful and meaningful, not only to him, but also to others. But to do so, he will need to spend more time with others to get a sense of what they need and want.

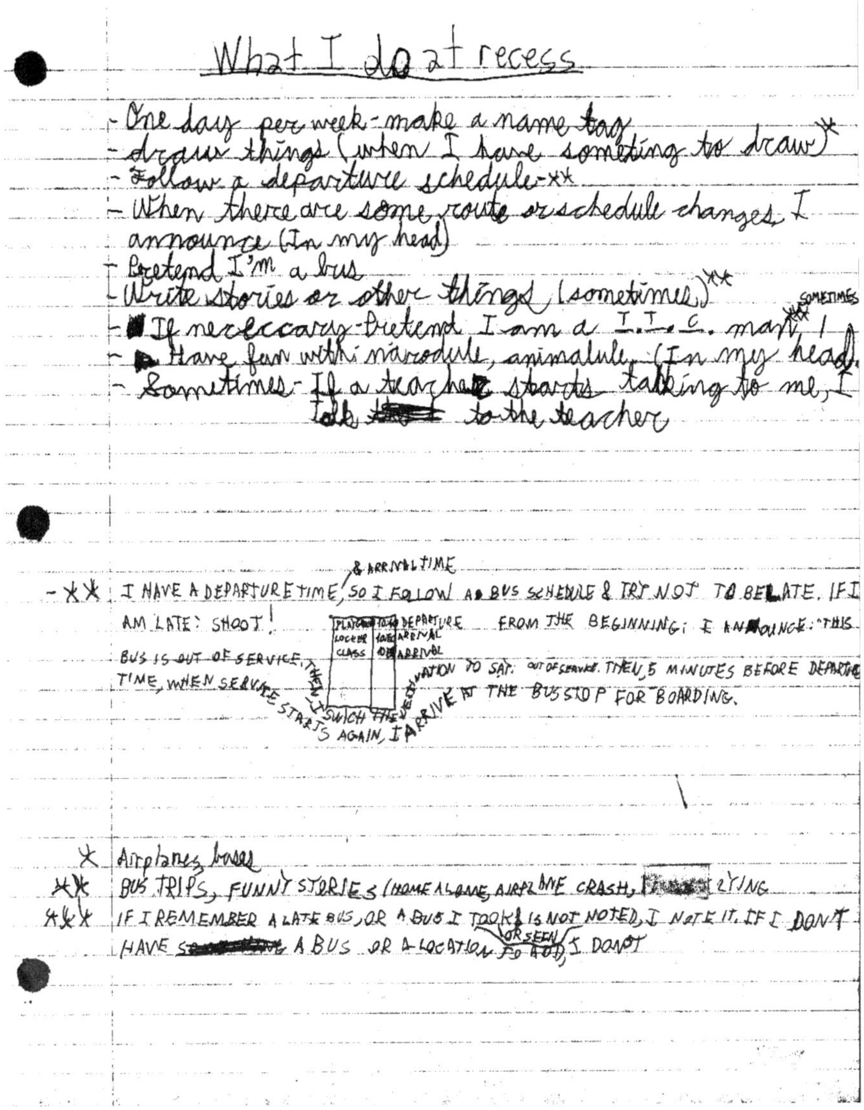
What I do at recess

- One day per week - make a name tag
- draw things (when I have something to draw)*
- Follow a departure schedule-**
- When there are some route or schedule changes I announce (In my head)
- Pretend I'm a bus
- Write stories or other things (sometimes)**
- If nececcary - pretend I am a I.T.C. man*** SOMETIMES !
- Have fun with narodule, animalule. (In my head)
- Sometimes - If a teacher starts talking to me, I talk [redacted] to the teacher

-** I HAVE A DEPARTURE TIME & ARRIVAL TIME, SO I FOLLOW A BUS SCHEDULE & TRY NOT TO BE LATE. IF I AM LATE: SHOOT! FROM THE BEGINNING: I ANNOUNCE: "THIS BUS IS OUT OF SERVICE." THEN I SWICH THE DESTINATION TO SAY: OUT OF SERVICE. THEN, 5 MINUTES BEFORE DEPARTURE TIME, WHEN SERVICE STARTS AGAIN, I ARRIVE AT THE BUS STOP FOR BOARDING.

PLACE	TO	DEPARTURE
LOCKER	LOCKER	ARRIVAL
CLASS	OR	ARRIVAL

* Airplanes, buses

** BUS TRIPS, FUNNY STORIES (HOME ALONE, AIRPLANE CRASH, [illegible] LYING

*** IF I REMEMBER A LATE BUS, OR A BUS I TOOK IS NOT NOTED, I NOTE IT. IF I DON'T HAVE [redacted] A BUS OR A LOCATION TO ADD OR SEEN, I DON'T

Figure 3.3: What I do at recess

4

An Autistic or Asperger Syndrome Child

The Scientific Perspective

So far we have learned about Teodor from those who know him the best: his family and school staff. Their knowledge of Teodor is based almost entirely on their own day-to-day experiences with Teodor as compared to his peers (or themselves when they were his age). Now let us consider Teodor from the perspectives of people who "know" many children like him. They provide a perspective on him in rather unnatural contexts, such as a laboratory or testing room. These perspectives, based on scientific methods of investigation, are supposed to help us get to know Teodor better than we can from everyday experience. In this chapter, we explore three perspectives on Teodor: psychiatric, psychological and neuroscientific.

Pervasive Developmental Disorder: The psychiatric perspective

> The patient is an 8-year-old boy with an early history of language delay, social withdrawal as well as focal obsessions, all beginning before 5 years of age. His obsessions with transportation routes and numbers to some extent have gone on for many years. He has developed some interest in other youngsters, but his interactive skills are clearly still weak. Cognitively, he appears to have a fair amount of strength, and he does not appear to be suffering from mental retardation. He has precocious puberty as well as the onset of epilepsy. From his history and his presentation today, it is clear that he has a diagnosis of Pervasive Developmental Disorder. The subtype is likely mild autism... If his obsessions and anxieties worsen, he may require pharmacological intervention. Luvox, Prozac or Paxil may be reasonable options...(Medical record of February 2, 1997)

When Teodor was eight years old (two weeks after the first story in this book took place) he had his first seizure episode and spent some time in a hospital. One of the doctors who treated him suggested that he be assessed by a psychiatrist. The above paragraph is the conclusion of this assessment. At a follow-up meeting, the psychiatrist told Teodor's parents that Teodor would be better described as having *Asperger's Disorder* rather than "mild autism." Accordingly, the diagnosis of Asperger's Disorder appears on all of Teodor's subsequent medical documents. Thus, his next medical record (dated eight months later, November 4, 1997), says that Teodor "meets the DSM-IV criteria for Asperger's Disorder" and "has Asperger's Disorder."

Two other parts of the psychiatrist's report help to understand the psychiatrist's diagnosis. The first part contains information about Teodor's development, obtained from his mother; the second part involves his observations and assessment of Teodor.

> ***Developmental history:*** The patient didn't start talking until he was about 2½–3 years of age. He only had a few words. When he began communicating, it was in short sentences. At around 3½ years of age, mother sent him to nursery school because he seemed as if he was in his "own world." He had little interest in terms of interacting with other children. He enjoyed affection and frequently initiated conversation with his family. At around 4 years of age, he became quite obsessed with bus routes and trams in Romania. He would memorize a whole variety of routes… When the patient came to Canada, he started in senior kindergarten. Of note, was the fact that he was already reading Romanian by 5 years of age. He was quite adept at numbers as well… He fidgets in the classroom, and has weird hand movements. He "hums and buzzes" in the classroom as well. His teacher says that he has "autistic like behaviors." In general, there were no major behaviour problems with the youngster up until last Summer. He went to day camp and was teased by other children. He started to lash out and hit kids. This continued on throughout the Fall. It has improved considerably since Christmas time…
>
> ***Individual assessment:*** The patient presents as an 8-year-old boy who was clearly very big for his age. He came in with his box of subway transfers. He began to go on and on about the various routes he took to get to the hospital. He had memorized the transfer numbers and some of the details on a piece of paper. He could recount the numbers on a previous transfer that he had taken over a year ago. Clearly, he was good with numbers, telling us the name of his phone number in Romania. He was living there almost 3 years ago. He would go on and on disregarding our general lack of interest in the area. His eye contact was reasonable, and his speech was somewhat high pitched. He related well to his mother, and he would

> frequently turn to her for hugs and affection. He told us a little bit about the kids that he plays with who clearly were much younger than him. He had trouble describing what they actually do together. His math and reading skills appeared to be basically age-appropriate, if not slightly above his level. His compre[hen]ssion [sic] is clearly weak.

When the psychiatrist diagnosed Teodor with mild autism/Asperger's Disorder, he also made two treatment recommendations: behavior management in a group of children with behavior problems (and their parents) and social skills training specifically designed for children diagnosed with Asperger's Disorder.

Commentary with explanations of terms

From the psychiatric report, we hear a very similar description of Teodor to that given by his family and the school staff, albeit from a very different perspective. We hear about the same kinds of behaviors, abilities, affections and conditions, including his difficulties in social interaction and communication, his "hobby" with public transit (now called an "obsession"), his fun with sounds (now called "humming and buzzing"), his high numerical and reading skills, but low reading comprehension skills, his affection towards his mother, and his precocious puberty which Teodor's father described as Teodor being "like a twelve-year-old with a sixteen-year-old body." Furthermore, the psychiatrist cautions that, if Teodor's "obsession" with public transit gets worse, it may need to be treated by medication.

We now also have some new information about Teodor. We learned about his developmental history, which includes relatively delayed language development, some restless and "weird" movements, incidences of aggressive behavior, anxiety and epilepsy.[12] The psychiatrist also used some new terms to describe Teodor: Pervasive Developmental Disorder, Asperger's Disorder, and mild autism. Let us first explain these terms, and then see how they relate to Teodor. This is fairly technical, so we ask forgiveness of our readers; but the detailed analysis that follows is critical to showing how children are assessed according to the scientific and clinical method. Those readers not interested in these technical details are invited to skip to the beginning of the next chapter.

The term *Pervasive Developmental Disorder* (PDD) is fairly new; it has only been in use by mental health professionals in North America since 1994. The term was created to refer to a set of mental disorders characterized by "impairments in social interaction, verbal and nonverbal communication", and "a repetitive pattern of behaviors" (American Psychiatric Association (APA) 1994). PPD is a general term that covers a family of five disorders: (1) Autistic Disorder;

(2) Asperger's Disorder; (3) Rett's Disorder; (4) Childhood Disintegrative Disorder; and (5) Pervasive Developmental Disorder Not Otherwise Specified. In Europe, the term "autistic spectrum disorder" is preferred over "Pervasive Developmental Disorder." Other terms, such as "autistic spectrum problems" (Gillberg 1990), "autism and autistic-like conditions" (Gillberg 1992) and "autistic continuum" (Wing 1988) have also been suggested as umbrella terms for these related conditions.

Today, in North America, *Autistic Disorder* (Kanner's autism,[13] or just plain autism) is a diagnosis given to those who meet specific criteria described in the *Diagnostic and Statistical Manual of Mental Disorders* DSM-IV (APA 1994) and DSM-IV-TR (APA 2000). Most other countries use similar criteria established by the World Health Organization (WHO) in the *ICD-10 International Classification of Diseases* (WHO 1992). The DSM-IV diagnostic criteria for Autistic Disorder require at least six "impairments" in areas of (1) social interaction, (2) communication, and (3) repetitive and stereotyped behavior and interests, as well as an onset of "delays or abnormal functioning" before the age of three (APA 1994, pp.70–71). The DSM-IV also lists several other features associated with Autistic Disorder such as unusual sensory and emotional responses, difficulty with attention, and behavior problems; however, none of these features are required for the diagnosis. (The full list of diagnostic criteria for Autistic Disorder can be found in Appendix B.)

A diagnosis of *Asperger's Disorder*[14] is given to individuals who meet specific diagnostic criteria, two of which are the same as for Autistic Disorder: impaired social interaction and repetitive behaviors/interests. However, instead of impairments in communication, which is critical to the diagnosis of Autistic Disorder, a diagnosis of Asperger's Disorder requires that there be "no clinically significant general delay in language" (APA 1994, p.77) and "no clinically significant delay in cognitive development or in the development of age-appropriate self-help skills, adaptive behavior (other than in social interaction), and curiosity about the environment in childhood" (p.77). However, there must be a "clinically significant impairment in social, occupational, or other important areas of functioning." Two additional associated features have been added for Asperger's Disorder: delayed motor milestones, and motor clumsiness. Finally, according to the DSM-IV, "Asperger's Disorder can be distinguished from Autistic Disorder by the lack of delay in language development" (APA 1994, p.69). (The full diagnostic criteria for Asperger's Disorder can be found in Appendix C.)

Now, after this barrage of definitions, we are in a better position to ask the key question: Does Teodor have mild Autistic Disorder or Asperger's Disorder, and does the difference matter?

According to the DSM-IV criteria, there should be at least two (out of four), characteristics present in Teodor's *social interaction* in order to make a diagnosis of Autistic Disorder. In Teodor's case, these two features could be: (1) "failure to develop peer relationships appropriate to developmental level," and (2) "lack of social or emotional reciprocity." The psychiatrist wrote that Teodor was able to tell him "a little bit about the kids that he plays with," that he plays with children who are "much younger than him," and that he has "trouble describing what they actually do together." These descriptions, together with descriptions obtained from Sandra about Teodor's developmental history—his lack of interest in interacting with other children, other children's teasing, and Teodor's subsequent aggressive outbursts—do fit these two characteristics. In addition, Teodor's family members also expressed concerns about Teodor's relationships with his peers, and mentioned somewhat better relationships with younger children and his lack of understanding reciprocity of friendship.

As for *communication*, only one characteristic is needed, and in fact, the psychiatrist emphasized Teodor's "early history of language delay" in his report. Another potential communication difficulty is Teodor's lack of "ability to initiate or sustain a conversation with others." The psychiatrist observed that Teodor "would go on and on [about the TTC routes he took on his way to the hospital] disregarding our general lack of interest in the area." Even though it is not clearly evident from the psychiatrist's report, another difficulty, "lack of varied, spontaneous make-believe play or social imitative play appropriate to developmental level," might be inferred from the fact that Sandra and Teodor did not talk to the psychiatrist about any make-believe play, nor was it mentioned in any family members' accounts of Teodor or by school staff. Another characteristic—"stereotyped and repetitive use of language or idiosyncratic language"—also applies to Teodor; we have seen examples of Teodor repeating words, sentences and conversations in the accounts of both parents and of the teaching assistant. However, it is not clear from the psychiatrist's report whether he was aware of all of this. Regardless, it is clear that Teodor's communication exhibits more than one of the characteristics required to diagnose autism.

Likewise, only one symptom from the area of "restricted repetitive and stereotyped patterns of behavior, interests, and activities" is needed for a diagnosis of autism. Clearly, Teodor's interest in public transit fits the description of "encompassing preoccupation with one or more stereotyped and restricted patterns of interest that is abnormal either in intensity or focus." The psychiatrist also noted that Teodor "has weird hand movements" which, if supported by more evidence, might be interpreted as "stereotyped and repetitive motor mannerism." Remember that in our introductory story about Teodor, we mentioned his jerking head movement that accompanied his "none-of-your-business" reply to other children who were curious about what he was doing. So this, too, might support the characterization of Teodor's behavior as "impaired" in this domain.

The diagnostic criteria require the presence of at least six characteristics from three domains for a diagnosis of autism to be made, at least one appearing before the age of three. According to the above analysis, there were more than the six required characteristics that applied to Teodor.

Considering the early beginning of the problems ("delays or abnormal functioning"), we learned from the psychiatrist's report that before the age of three Teodor had "little interest in terms of interacting with other children"; thus, Teodor meets the requirement for early onset of "abnormal functioning" in social interaction. The psychiatrist also wrote that Teodor "didn't start talking until he was about 2½–3 years of age," and concluded that he had "early history of language delay," a second area of interest. Also, Teodor's mother pointed out that Teodor was also delayed in a third domain relevant for the diagnosis, "symbolic or imaginative play," which he also did not engage in before the age of three. So it seems that Teodor's early development has been characterized by delays in at least two of the domains listed as critical for a diagnosis of autism, which is more than sufficient.

Finally, from the diagnostic point of view it is critical that Teodor's problems were not better accounted for by *Rett's Disorder* or *Childhood Disintegrative Disorder* (both of which are characterized by a sudden deterioration in functioning).

So all in all, Teodor clearly fulfills the DSM-IV diagnostic criteria for Autistic Disorder. But in his report, the psychiatrist suggested that Teodor has "mild autism." However, DSM-IV does not specify any further distinctions within Autistic Disorder. It only acknowledges the existence of differences in the level of functioning related to general intellectual abilities of those diagnosed with Autistic Disorder. We find the term "higher functioning" to refer to those who "function" outside a retarded level. Teodor's psychiatrist probably found Teodor's autism to be "mild" because Teodor did "not appear to be suffering from mental retardation." In the scientific literature on autism, the term "high-functioning autism" is used synonymously with "mild autism."

Now that it is clearer what the psychiatrist might have meant when he said that Teodor is "mildly autistic," let us see why he might have changed his mind and said that Teodor has Asperger's Disorder by examining how the DSM-IV diagnostic criteria for this disorder relate to Teodor.

According to the DSM-IV guidelines for differential diagnosis, "Asperger's Disorder is not diagnosed if criteria are met for Autistic Disorder" (p.69)—the so-called "precedence rule." Teodor did meet them, so technically he does not qualify for the DSM-IV Asperger's label. However, there is more to this label (or perhaps less) than we find in the current DSM-IV criteria. In the literature on Asperger's Disorder, we consistently find that clinicians and researchers do not apply the DSM-IV rules very strictly. In fact, some recent studies have suggested that, if applied strictly, DSM-IV criteria for the diagnosis of Asperger's Disorder may not apply to anybody (Eisenmajer *et al.* 1996; Mayes, Calhoun and Crites 2001)—not even the children described by Hans Asperger (Miller and Ozonoff 1997)! This is because the current diagnostic requirement is that the diagnosis of Asperger's Disorder should not be made if the criteria for Autistic Disorder are met; all four cases described by Asperger met these criteria—as did Teodor.

Teodor's psychiatrist judged that Teodor had language delay. Since the DSM-IV criteria require the absence of "clinically significant delay" in *language development* for the diagnosis of Asperger's Disorder (defined as the use of single words by the age of two, and communicative phrases by the age of three), Teodor should not have been given the diagnosis of Asperger's Disorder. However, many clinicians and researchers believe that the presence of language delay does not preclude a diagnosis of Asperger's Disorder (e.g., Eisenmajer *et al.* 1996; Gillberg 1989, 1991, 2002;[15] Tantam 1991; Wing 1981). Moreover, two out of the four cases described by Asperger (1944/1991) had language delay. Psychiatrist Christopher Gillberg recently suggested that

> Maybe one in three of all children with Asperger syndrome do not speak at all or only very little around age 3 years. It is common for expressive language to develop at an almost explosive rate during the next one or two years. From having said virtually nothing at age 3, the child may well be able to speak in long and complicated sentences only a few months later. (2002, p.28)

This pattern clearly resembles Teodor's. According to his mother, Teodor "didn't start talking until he was about 2½–3 years of age. He only had a few words. When he began communicating, it was in short sentences."

Richard Eisenmajer and his colleagues (1996) reported that almost half (43%) of the children with Asperger syndrome in their study had some kind of language delay. Moreover, researchers stress the difficulty of establishing the existence of a delay since in most cases the evidence about it is retrospective (Howlin 2003). In Teodor's case, evidence about his early language development is based on his mother's recollection of events that took place 5–6 years earlier. According to her recollection, Teodor started talking when he was "about 2½–3."

It is ironic that, after all of this effort at distinguishing Asperger's Disorder from high-functioning autism (Autistic Disorder), many experts believe that there is no difference between them, and that the former is just a mild variant of the latter (Schopler 1996, 1998; Wing 1988, 2000) or that Asperger's Disorder is just a later developmental expression of Autistic Disorder (Attwood 1998; Szatmari 2000).

Lorna Wing (1988) has argued that these two conditions are on the same continuum (i.e., they differ only in degrees of social and cognitive impairments) and that there are no qualitative differences between them, as is suggested by DSM-IV. Moreover, she maintains that in her 1981 paper in which she used the term Asperger syndrome, she only intended to suggest that this condition might be on a continuum with the condition Leo Kanner described, not that it is a different and easily separable disorder (2000). She further believes that the cases in which the "same individual was typically autistic in his early years but made progress and as a teenager showed all characteristics of Asperger's syndrome [are] the strongest argument for a seamless continuum from Kanner autism to Asperger's syndrome" (1991, p.103). Similarly, Tony Attwood (1998) suggests that both diagnoses could be given to the same child at different points in time as in cases where the "previous diagnosis of classic autism was accurate when the child was very young, but the child has progressed along the autistic continuum to the expression we call Asperger's Syndrome" (p.23). Moreover, he argues "it is essential that the diagnosis of autism is regularly reviewed to examine whether Asperger's Syndrome is now a more accurate diagnosis" (pp.23–4). Peter Szatmari (2000) too views Asperger's Disorder as a developmental progression of Autistic Disorder. He contends that these two conditions are not different biological entities, but rather two different developmental pathways that could be differentiated on the basis of language acquisition by three years of age. According to him, children who develop fluent language by this age follow Asperger's trajectory, whilst children who do not, follow an autistic trajectory. However, if the child on the autistic trajectory develops language, he or she will move to the Asperger trajectory. In fact, we find many reports in the literature about children who met the criteria for Autistic Disorder in their pre-school years, but later appeared to be cases of Asperger's Disorder in their school-age years or in adulthood (Gillberg 1989, 1991, 2002; Tantam 1991; Wing 1981, 1988, 1991). Teodor, then, might have appeared to the psychiatrist as a case of Autistic Disorder retrospectively, but he might have better resembled a case of Asperger's Disorder at the time of the diagnosis.

On that note, it remains open as to why Teodor's psychiatrist felt that Teodor is better described as Asperger's than autistic, and indeed many other clinicians might have made a similar "shift." In fact, after six decades since its first description, issues of definition are still a major concern in clinical diagnosis and on research on Asperger syndrome (Blacher, Kraemer and Schalow 2003).

Reflections

Why diagnose? You may have noticed that none of Teodor's family members mentioned autism in their descriptions of him. This is particularly interesting in light of his parents' knowledge of this condition, or disorder. Both Sandra and Andrew have met or seen videos about autistic children and adults, in addition to what they learned from the psychiatrist. Sandra had also read a number of books and articles about autism, and has participated in a few workshops on the topic. We believe that this "omission" suggests that they do not find the term "autistic" very descriptive of Teodor as a person, or as a member of their family. An autistic person, Liane Holliday Willey, recently wrote that her friend (who understands and accepts her the way she is) sees her "*first* as someone who possesses many good qualities, and only then as someone who is just a tiny bit different" (1999, p.73). This is how Teodor's family members see Teodor, too—as a person with good qualities, but a little bit different.

Interestingly enough, the school staff did not use the term autistic in their descriptions of Teodor, either. Now, is it fair to say that since Teodor's family members and school staff did not mention autism, that it doesn't matter to them whether or not Teodor is autistic? The truth is that if it hadn't been for this diagnosis, Teodor would not have been given a teaching assistant, and his English instruction might not have been modified to accommodate his low reading comprehension skills. However, the quality of the help he received in school was not in any way intended to remediate his "core autistic deficits." Teodor received no help regarding his "impairments" in social interaction, communication and stereotyped interest/behaviors. Rather, the help he received was aimed at improving his academic achievement. But the success of autistic individuals later in life depends crucially not on their level of education but on their level of social competence (Howlin 2003; Klin and Volkmar 2000). Thus, the school's single-minded focus on academic achievement is not defensible. Adults with high-functioning autism or Asperger syndrome have low employment status in spite of high education (Howlin 2003). As Klin and Volkmar remark, "Many adults with this condition are not given an opportunity to exhibit their considerable talents and skills because of failure during the interview stage of job applications" (2000, p.350).

Moreover, by not helping Teodor develop his social competences, his school fails to prevent some common consequences of an inability to fit in, usually referred to as "secondary psychological disorders" such as affective disorders and conduct disorders, which might further impede both social and educational progress. Recent findings show that these disorders are indeed common among autistic children and adolescents (Green *et al.* 2000; Howlin 2003; Kim *et al.* 2000; Tantam 2000b; Tonge *et al.* 1999).

Finally, educational accommodations for Teodor's difficulties with language comprehension through more time to complete the assignments and reading material at a lower grade level do not take the reasons for Teodor's reading comprehension difficulty into account. Nor do they consider Teodor's specific "autistic" learning style (e.g., visual and experiential) or use any specific teaching strategy to help remediate his learning difficulties (see Klin and Volkmar 2000; Quill 1995). Therefore, Teodor was not given the sort of specific "exceptional educational treatment" advocated by Asperger (1944/1991, p.37). (The reader interested in educational issues in Asperger's Disorder is referred to recent reviews and guidelines by Klin and Volkmar 2000; Kunce and Mesibov 1998; National Research Council (US) Committee on Educational Interventions for Children with Autism 2001; and Prior 2003).

Perhaps because, at present, the school system has not yet been held responsible for implementing the social skills component of the special educational program for autistic children, the psychiatrist also recommended that Teodor participate in an intervention specifically designed to remediate social deficit in children diagnosed with Asperger's Disorder—social skills training. However, this intervention did not meet parental expectations of what help their son needed the most—improved social interaction and communication *with children*, and especially at the playground. Instead, the skills he was taught resembled rote skills of polite behavior with adults—in which Teodor was pretty skilled already.[16] This parental observation echoes Patricia Howlin's view that, "Teaching new skills, or correcting errors *in situ*, is far more likely to be effective than teaching in the relative isolation of a 'social skills group'" (1998, p.161).

Others too have emphasized the importance (and showed the effectiveness) of learning social skills in naturalistic contexts (Broderick *et al.* 2002; Paul 2003; Whitaker *et al.* 1998), and peer-mediated social skills training and peer social interaction-tutoring (Rogers 2000).[17] Moreover, some studies have shown that skills learned in social skills training do not generalize to other settings (e.g., Barnhill *et al.* 2002; Ozonoff and Miller 1995). From his extensive clinical experience, psychotherapist and psychiatrist Digby Tantam notes that children who had social contacts with peers improved more over the years than those who did not. He suggested that the key element of this improvement might be the "social demand that is associated with peer interaction: Peers do not make explicit demands, but they also make few allowances" (Tantam 2003).

We agree: school *is* where social skills should be taught, among—and *by*—children and in real situations, not in artificial settings through "prototypical examples" explained by adults and practiced by rote. Examples of this kind of intervention involving peers include peer-mediated social skills training (Kamps *et al.* 2002; Pierce and Schreibman 1995, 1997) and "circle of friends" (Whitaker *et al.* 1998). But Teodor's school failed to provide not only the most effective peer-mediated social skills intervention, but also any intervention that targets his core difficulty in social learning.[18]

Autistic or Asperger's Disorder? For Teodor's family and school it does not really seem to matter whether Teodor has Autistic or Asperger's Disorder. Moreover, it does not even seem to matter whether Teodor has autism or not. He is treated with the same care and respect that he would receive if he did not have any of these labels. It would, of course, be important to distinguish between Autistic and Asperger's Disorder if different treatment options existed for these two conditions—but they do not. Therefore, this issue does not have any apparent practical relevance—at least not at the moment, although if Teodor were not diagnosed at all, that would make a difference. However, from a theoretical perspective, the difference between Autistic and Asperger's Disorder is an important one. But, in order to determine whether there is a real difference between Autistic and Asperger's Disorders, we must be able to distinguish them in terms of their causes, specific patterns of brain involvement, and performance on psychological, physiological, motor or any other tasks. The ultimate aim of such a distinction is to develop different treatments for these two conditions—if they exist.

In fact, Teodor's case is a good example of what happens when there is a professional confusion regarding diagnostic criteria—not only might two diagnosticians hypothetically give Teodor different diagnoses, but he was actually given two different diagnoses by the same diagnostician, at two different points in time. Moreover, if chosen as a subject for a scientific study, he might be considered a case of autism in one, and a case of Asperger's Disorder in another. This is a big research problem as many studies are concerned precisely with the question of whether there is a difference between these two conditions or not. A recent systematic review of the literature over the past 15 years identified 26 studies (published in major journals) that dealt with this issue (Howlin 2003). But we must ask ourselves how meaningful the results of these studies could be if the same subject could belong to both investigating conditions. Also, the disagreements in the diagnostic criteria make cross-study comparisons impossible because subjects considered to have Asperger syndrome in one study, because they did not have language delay, can be considered as autistic in another (see Volkmar and Klin 2000).

Not only that, the current DSM-IV diagnostic criteria may be said to contribute to important omissions in the diagnosticians' reports about autistic persons. For example, there is something important missing in the psychiatrist's description of Teodor. Teodor has a characteristic—stiff and rather awkward—gait that would make him stick out in a group of people walking, running or jumping. It is the kind of gait that could help you recognize him in a crowd, from behind, or from afar. In fact, when Teodor was in Grade 3, his teacher requested occupational therapy assessment and consultation "with regard to his gross motor skills affecting his gym program." The occupational therapist concluded that Teodor:

> appears to have a gross motor clumsiness or awkwardness during certain physical activities (i.e., running, jumping). (Summary of the occupational therapist's assessment, June, 1998)

Both Hans Asperger and Ewa Ssucharewa observed awkward gait in children they described. But in spite of being recognized by Asperger (1944/1991) as a core characteristic of the condition he identified, motor clumsiness is not included among the core impairments of Asperger's Disorder in the DSM-IV; instead, it is listed as an "associated" feature. And since, "we find what we are prepared to find (what we look for or what forcefully affronts our expectations), and...are likely to be blind to what neither helps nor hinders our pursuits" (Goodman 1978, p.22), this psychiatrist, who was not "prepared to find" anything special about Teodor's movements, did not pay any attention to, nor record, anything about them.

However, we think that a "small" detail such as the way Teodor came into the psychiatrist's office is very important from the theoretical perspective and might eventually turn out to have practical consequences. In spite of contradictory findings[19] about the existence of movement impairments in Asperger's Disorder (or perhaps because of these contradictions),[20] we believe that mental health professionals should record them. In fact, they should record anything out of the ordinary in these patients, regardless of the current diagnostic criteria—in particular, characteristics like motor clumsiness that were found in previous reports. More detailed records are particularly important in these cases since, as we have seen, our current diagnostic categories are not satisfactory and we need unbiased descriptions in order to create better ones. In fact, many clinicians and researchers often use other, unofficial, diagnostic criteria, such as ones proposed by Christopher Gillberg (1991), which include *motor clumsiness* as an essential characteristic.

Similarly, in Teodor's medical record we find no data on his *sensory functioning.* Again, in Asperger's (1944/1991) original report we find descriptions of sensory peculiarities such as hypo- and hypersensitivities to auditory, tactile, and taste, but not visual, stimuli. (For recent reviews of characteristics of sensory processing in Asperger syndrome see Dunn, Saiter and Rinner 2002; and Myles *et al.* 2000.) Again, it is easy to imagine that these "other characteristics" or "associated features" such as motor and sensory characteristics may hold a key to the progress in distinguishing between Autistic and Asperger's Disorder. They may be crucial in discovering fundamental mechanisms underlying these disorders. Moreover, once we have a more precise knowledge about all the characteristics of these conditions and their developmental trajectories, this distinction might have important practical implications for early identification, and condition-specific intervention.

After this long and complex discussion about the many uncertainties associated with Asperger syndrome, why include "Asperger syndrome" in the book subtitle when its very existence has not yet been established? We have two reasons: First, Teodor better resembles cases described by Hans Asperger, Gillberg, Ssucharewa and Wing than those described by Leo Kanner. In particular, Teodor's motor characteristics and unusual interest in public transit fit better into Asperger syndrome category. Consequently, we use the unofficial label Asperger syndrome, instead of DSM-IV label Asperger's Disorder.[21] Second, we have seen many autistic and Asperger syndrome children and *feel* that there is *something* different about them, in spite of many similarities—a difference that has so far been difficult to pinpoint. It may be that only when we look at autistic children and adults as persons, will we find this subtle qualitative difference, which may prove to be beyond the ability of our formal assessment instruments to capture (a point not unlike that made by Katherine Tsatsanis (2003)). Finally, it is worth remembering that after many years of working with autistic children—and after reading Leo Kanner's paper—Hans Asperger still felt that children Kanner and he described in the 1940s were "basically different types" (1979, p.47).

"Mind-blind": The psychological perspective

Let us now see what psychology—another scientific discipline that concerns itself with persons and their minds—has to offer in our effort to understand Teodor. In this section we will present the psychometric, cognitive and developmental perspectives on Teodor.

Autistic intelligence: The psychometric perspective

> The results of the WISC-III indicate that Teodor's reasoning abilities are developing slowly. His overall score fell within the Borderline range at the

> 2nd percentile.[22] He shows weaknesses in both the verbal and non-verbal domains. His score of verbal abilities fell in the Borderline range at the 7th percentile. His score of non-verbal abilities fell in the Intellectually Deficient range at the 2nd percentile.
>
> These results should be considered within the context of Teodor's Pervasive Developmental Disorder diagnosis.
>
> Due to motivational and English-as-a-second-language (ESL) factors, these test results may underestimate Teodor's cognitive functioning. (WISC-III: Conclusion, August 2, 2001)

The psychiatrist who diagnosed Teodor as having Autistic Disorder suggested that Teodor "appears to have a fair amount of strength, and he does not appear to be suffering from mental retardation," but suggested Teodor's intelligence be tested. An intelligence test was not administered to Teodor at that time; however, in order to obtain a more complete account of Teodor, Ljiljana, under the supervision of a clinical psychologist, Nancy Link,[23] conducted the testing with the Wechsler Intelligence Scale for Children—Third Edition (WISC-III) when Teodor was twelve years old. The WISC-III is a widely used intelligence test for children between six and sixteen years old. It consists of many questions and tasks grouped into two scales, verbal and nonverbal (i.e., performance), and each containing five subtests. The scores from these subtests are summed into three measures of intelligence (intelligence quotients): verbal, performance and total IQs. (This test also contains two "supplementary" subtests—Digit Span and Mazes—whose scores are not calculated into the overall score.) The opening excerpt for this chapter is the conclusion of the WISC-III intelligence test report. The full report includes details about Teodor's performance on individual subtests:

> He showed particular strength (well above average) in his ability to remember a series of numbers (Digit Span). He showed relative strength in his ability to perform mental arithmetic calculations (Arithmetic). He showed particular weakness in his knowledge of interpersonal relations and social mores (Comprehension).
>
> Teodor's nonverbal abilities fell within the Intellectually Deficient range, at the 2nd percentile. He showed relative strength on a task requiring visualization and planning (Mazes). He showed relative weakness on a task requiring putting puzzle pieces together to make a whole object (Object Assembly). He also showed relative weakness on a task requiring that he notice missing details in a picture (Picture Completion).

Interestingly, Digit Span and Mazes—the "supplementary" subtests—are where Teodor obtained his highest scores. The Digit Span subtest is said to "measure" short-term auditory memory, while the Mazes subtest measures visuospatial abilities. On the Mazes subtest his score fell into the "average" range, while on the Digit Span subtest his score actually fell in the "superior" range. Furthermore, the subject's level of motivation and attention during the testing are important to consider when interpreting intelligence test results:

> Even though, in general, Teodor listened to instructions, he had difficulty understanding 'work-as-fast-as-you-can' instructions. On these tasks he adopted a rather playful approach and did not seem to understand that it was important to try to work quickly. For example, after I realized that Teodor is not trying to work as fast as he can, on the next task I emphasized the instruction that he should do so by the change in my voice.[24] Teodor noticed the change in my voice, and began to have fun repeating "work-as-fast-as-you-can"—in my voice. In addition, after he would finish a task in which he also needed to indicate when he is done, he would do so by inventing "funny" things: he would spell "D-O-N-E," arrange the pictures so they look "funny" and so on. (Excerpt from Observation Notes)

Reflections

What do these results mean? As the psychiatrist suggested, Teodor's results on the WISC-III indicate that he is not mentally retarded. However, the test results suggest that he borders on being mentally retarded. In fact, he is within a few points of the boundary. But, what exactly do Teodor's results on the WISC-III tell us about Teodor's intelligence, Teodor's autism—or Teodor himself?

Teodor's mother's first reaction to the results of his WISC-III intelligence test is the best answer to the question of what these results *mean*. She said, "Now we know Teodor is not good on this kind of test." But what is "this kind of test"? According to current theorizing about intelligence testing, the WISC-III really tests only a small portion of intellectual abilities—analytical abilities—and not even all of them (Sattler 1992; Sternberg 1986, 2000). According to psychologist Robert Sternberg (1986), in addition to analytical abilities there are also creative and practical intellectual abilities that are not addressed by these tests. Other scholars too have suggested that there are more than one type of intelligence. Psychologist Howard Gardner (1993, 1998), for example, has recently suggested that there are at least eight or nine intelligences: linguistic, logical-mathematical, spatial, musical, bodily-kinesthetic, natural (understanding nature), interpersonal (i.e., understanding and interacting with others), and intrapersonal (i.e., understanding oneself) and possibly existential. According to those who believe in multiple intelligences, the fact that Teodor did not do very well on a psychometric intelligence test tells us next to nothing about his intellectual abilities overall. To get a more "realistic" portrait of Teodor's intelligence, his other abilities should be assessed. Moreover, Gardner does not agree that standardized tests are the right way to approach the assessment of any intellectual ability—instead he argues that observation and analysis of cultural products and performance on tasks that require a specific ability are better forms of assessment.

We agree. Here is why.

The Mazes subtest on the WISC-III is designed to measure visuospatial abilities—which parallels "spatial intelligence" in Gardner's taxonomy. But, although Teodor obtained an average score on this subtest, in real life his abilities in this domain seem higher than average. He orients himself remarkably well in

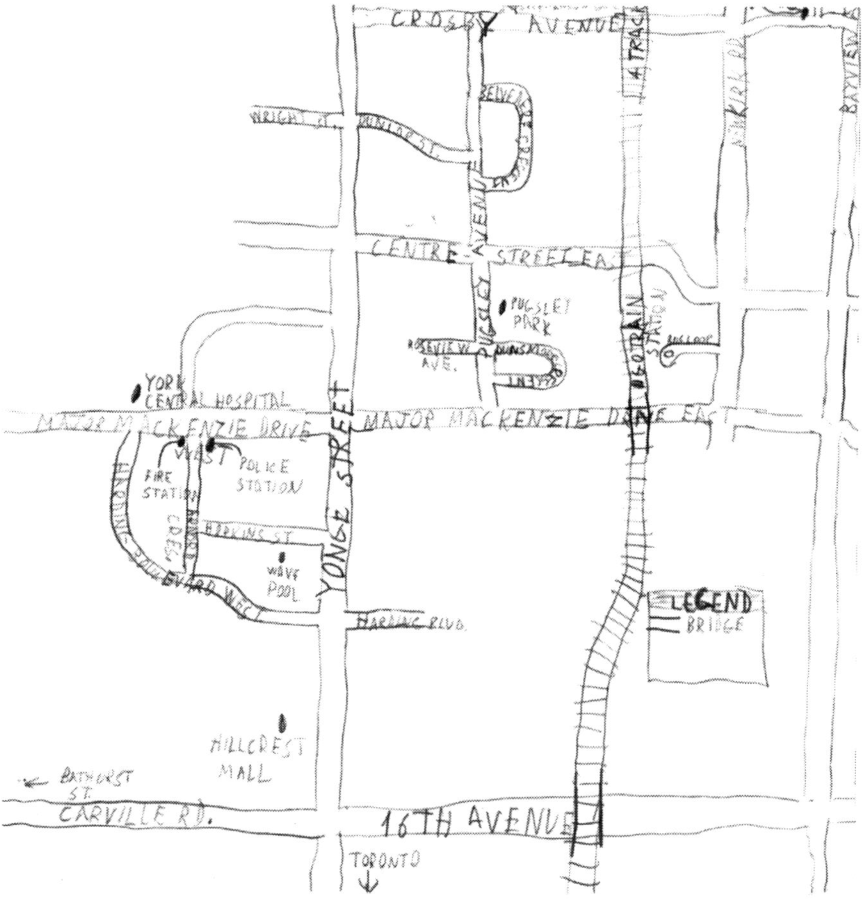

Figure 4.1: Teodor's map drawing

space and has an exceptional memory for spatial relations; he can also represent these relations in drawings (Figure 4.1) or three-dimensional models on an above-average level (Figures 4.2 and 4.3).

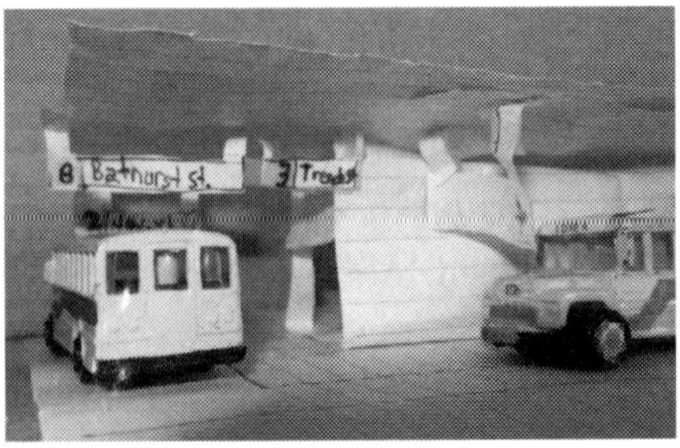

Figure 4.2: The outside of Teodor's paper model of a bus station

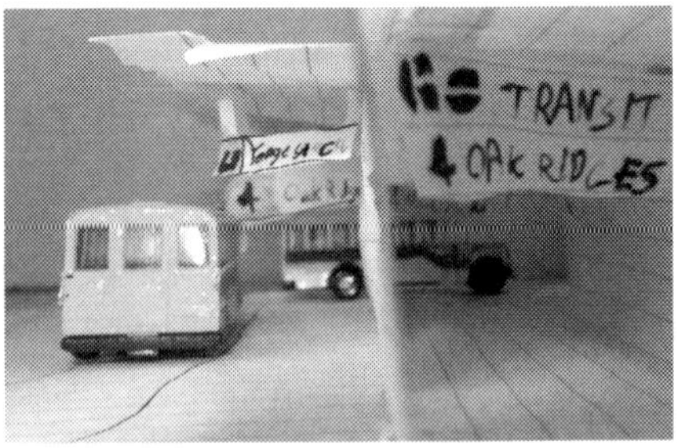

Figure 4.3: Another look at Teodor's bus station model

In addition, many researchers and clinicians (including Asperger himself) have questioned the suitability of using standardized testing with autistic children. As Alan Lincoln, Mark Allen and Angela Kilman (1995) suggested, "Any item a[n autistic] child can pass during formal psychometric assessment is probably a real sample of their ability. However, the opposite is not true" (p.110).[25] There are many factors besides ability that are needed in order to succeed on a task (e.g., motivation and attention). Therefore, as Alan Lincoln and his colleagues suggest, a much better index of intellectual abilities in autistic persons is obtained by closely examining their functioning "in context[s] where their motivation and attention may be much higher" (p.111). Here is another example of how this applies to Teodor.

One question on the test asked what to do when someone cuts her or his finger. Teodor said, "Put a glove so it does not show it's cut." Ljiljana was surprised by this answer since she knew that Teodor knew the correct answer. Since the intelligence testing does not allow for the probing of an answer, that was his final—obviously wrong—answer. This subtest is the one on which Teodor scored at the mentally retarded level.

And yet a few weeks later, when Ljiljana visited Teodor at his home, she and Sandra prepared the following scene: Sandra and Ljiljana were sitting on the porch, while Teodor was inside the house. Sandra pretended that she had cut her finger and Ljiljana called Teodor and asked him what he should do. He immediately said that he needed to go and get the band-aids, and he went right away. He came back with them a few minutes later (without asking anybody where they were), opened the wrapping and wanted to apply the band-aid to his mother's finger—the plot was then revealed to him. When Ljiljana asked him why he told her in the testing room that one should cover it, he said that he understood the question was about cutting a finger *off*, and that he recently saw in a movie (*Mighty Joe Young*) that somebody put a glove on when that happened. Moreover, as you may remember, in providing an example of Teodor's "understanding of others," Teodor's mother said, "If a friend is hurt, he would try to help—he would come home, get the band-aid, go there, take care, and just try to help."[26] This is why we join Lincoln, Allen and Kilman (1995) in their call for rethinking our approach to intelligence testing in autistic individuals.

This example illustrates how observation of Teodor's performance in everyday life is a better test of his intelligence than the WISC-III. This is true of everyone (Gardner 1993, 1998; Sternberg 1997; Sternberg and Wagner 1994), but it applies especially to autistic children (and to other "kinds" of atypical children). As we have seen, Teodor did not correctly answer the question for which he "knew" the answer. Besides, Teodor's mother suggested that he perhaps did not try "his best" because he did not take the test seriously enough, since Ljiljana used the word "special activities" and not "test" when she explained what they were doing. Teodor takes tests much more seriously than "activities" regardless of the instruction to do "as best as you can." This additional information is supported by Teodor's numerous attempts to have fun during the testing. All these examples illustrate that such tests are not the best way to obtain a realistic portrait of Teodor's abilities. Ecologically valid measures are more appropriate. And although some researchers have suggested that autistic children usually function much better in the test situation because it is more structured than the real world (Szatmari 2000), Teodor's case certainly does not support this view.

In spite of their theoretical and methodological problems, standardized tests of intelligence remain the most common way of evaluating the intellectual functioning of autistic persons, both clinically and in research. Most clinicians and researchers agree that autistic persons display specific patterns of deficits and strengths on standardized tests of intelligence (Asperger 1944/1991; Green *et al.* 1995; Kanner 1943; Sandberg *et al.* 1993; Szatmari *et al.* 1990; Wing 1981); however, there is no consensus on what exactly this profile is. A peak score on the Block Design subtest has commonly been reported (Ehlers *et al.* 1997; Happé 1994b; Lincoln *et al.* 1995), but other patterns of performance have also been found (e.g., Ozonoff, South and Miller 2000). For a recent review of cognitive profiles of children and youth diagnosed with autism and Asperger's Disorder obtained from the Wechsler scales, see Barnhill *et al.* (2000).

Some researchers suggest that children with Asperger's Disorder have different cognitive profiles than do children diagnosed with Autistic Disorder, and that these profiles can be used to distinguish between these two disorders (Klin *et al.* 1995; Lincoln *et al.* 1998). However, the evidence so far has been mixed; for example, some studies have found that children with Asperger's Disorder have higher verbal than performance IQ, while autistic children show the opposite pattern (Klin *et al.* 1995; Lincoln *et al.* 1998; Miller and Ozonoff 2000); but not all studies confirm this finding (Manjiviona and Prior 1999; Ozonoff *et al.* 2000). For example, a recent study examining the performance of children with Asperger's Disorder and high-functioning autism (which used strict DSM-IV criteria to assigning subjects to groups), found that 50 per cent of children with Asperger's Disorder performed better on verbal tasks, while 8 per cent of them had the opposite pattern (Ozonoff *et al.* 2000).[27] In the same study, 35 per cent of children diagnosed with high-functioning autism also had better performance on verbal tasks, while 17 per cent of them had the opposite pattern. These differences between the two groups of autistic participants were not statistically significant.

Another common view of children with Asperger's Disorder's "typical pattern" of performance on the WISC-III is the lower score on the Comprehension subtest relative to the Block Design subtest (Lincoln *et al.* 1998). However, some studies also found that children with Asperger's Disorder performed well on the Comprehension subtest (obtaining one of the highest scores of the verbal subtest on it; Ozonoff *et al.* 2000).

Given the previously discussed ambiguity of diagnostic criteria, these inconsistent results are not surprising. The fact that most studies found that children with Asperger's Disorder have higher verbal abilities than children with Autistic Disorder is also not surprising, since the diagnostic criteria themselves require an absence of language delay for the diagnosis of Asperger's Disorder. It is worth mentioning that Teodor's profile fits into this generalization, as he obtained a higher score for his verbal as compared to his nonverbal task performances.

Asperger himself noted that, "[j]ust as, in general, somebody's good and bad sides are inextricably linked, so the *special abilities and disabilities* of autistic people are interwoven" (1944/1991, p.70; our emphasis). However, in both research and education in the field of autism, the positive end of the ability spectrum has been largely neglected. Although there have been some recent attempts to correct this negativity bias in studying intellectual abilities in autism (Happé 1994a,

1999a, b; Shah and Frith 1993), research still emphasizes deficits. Similarly, in educational contexts, some autistic and Asperger syndrome children are recognized as twice-exceptional learners (i.e., as possessing a unique combination of giftedness and disability; Cash 1999; Little 2002; Yewchuk and Lupart 2000). However, *all* children with Asperger syndrome possess characteristics of giftedness as commonly defined (i.e., high ability in one or more areas of human activity, intense interest and focus in area of high ability, as well as *precocity*—earlier than average acquisition of skills or knowledge and faster than average learning in some areas; Winner 1998). As such, we believe, all children with Asperger syndrome should receive educational support in the specific areas of their giftedness and not only in the area of their deficit.

Asperger also believed that the special abilities of autistic children "can *in favorable cases* lead to exceptional achievements which others may never attain" (1944/1991, p.74; our emphasis). He underlined autistic children's "potential value to society" (p.87) provided they receive the appropriate education and guidance. However, despite the success of some autistic individuals at becoming respected experts in their fields, such individuals are more an exception than the rule. Temple Grandin's autobiography (Grandin and Scariano 1986) clearly testifies to how crucial educational guidance and support are in transforming the "potential" of autistic individuals into the real value to society of which Asperger spoke. In her case, there was somebody—her teacher—who believed in "building what was within the student" (p.82), and who channeled her exceptional spatial abilities and "fixations into constructive projects" (p.82) which led her to become a respectful livestock facility designer. Unfortunately, Teodor's case is an example, more common, of inadequate educational support: No attention has been paid to any of his special abilities—neither those identified through the intelligence test (i.e., spatial and numerical), nor those he exhibits in everyday-life situations (i.e., visual-spatial and sound imitation). Teodor's "special gift" at sound imitation, for example, is usually talked about as his "bad habit;" instead of being developed in a constructive way through drama classes, it is viewed as odd and either punished or ignored.

Finally, what to make of Teodor's WISC-III results, which indicate that his intellectual abilities border on mental retardation, in light of the general agreement among psychologists and psychiatrists that intelligence scores in both typical and atypical (including autistic) populations have good predictive value (i.e., predict school success, job performance and overall well-being; Frith 1991; Howlin *et al.* 2004; Rutter, Greenfeld and Lockyer 1967; Sternberg, Grigorenko and Bundy 2001). It is important to bear in mind that Teodor's profile of abilities is uneven (i.e., his abilities span a range from mental retardation—on the task that measures understanding of social rules—to the superior level for numerical memory). We believe that his composite score tells us nothing about his specific intellectual potentials, nor about his prognosis in real-life situations. The same holds true, we believe, for assessment of any individual with a highly uneven profile of intellectual abilities. Not only that, as Robert Sternberg and his colleagues (2001) warn, other factors influence school and life success besides the analytic intelligences measured on psychometric tests, such as parental or other caregivers' support.

Therefore, the label of "borderline intelligence" is neither appropriate nor informative when classifying or describing individuals like Teodor, who have an uneven profile of abilities and a great deal of parental support. In fact, together with Hans Asperger, we believe that "autistic intelligence" is of a different kind and requires a different kind of assessment and a different kind of support than intelligence of typically developing children. And, as Asperger observed, even autistic children with "borderline intelligence" can succeed in school (provided schoolwork capitalizes on their strengths and compensates for their weaknesses), have fulfilling careers, and live happy and productive lives.

Autistic mind: The cognitive and developmental perspectives

THE SEARCH FOR CORE DEFICITS

The current research practice for studying autism in psychology involves studying isolated aspects of autism (i.e., dependent variables) and "controlling for" a certain number of "confounding" factors (e.g., intelligence, language, sex, or age). The aim of such studies is to test for specific hypotheses that explain the statistical difference (the variance) between the performance of autistic subjects and that of other individuals—control subjects—either typical individuals or other types of atypical individuals, such as mentally retarded individuals, or individuals with attention deficit hyperactivity disorder, conduct disorders, or William's syndrome. The way a disorder is conceptualized influences the sort of characteristics examined and the methods used.

We will briefly review some of the major theoretical perspectives from cognitive psychology and the main findings from the research inspired by them. For the past forty years,[28] psychological science has attempted to explain autism (and, more recently, Asperger syndrome) in ways very much characterized by the search for core deficits that could explain all other features of autism as "secondary reactions to the primary problems" (Frith 1991, p.17). These attempts have adopted the prevailing psychological theories and methods of their time—including learning theory, information-processing theory and Theory of Mind. Within these various approaches, researchers have singled out almost every psychological function (e.g., emotions, attention, language, memory, executive functions) as the most crucial to explaining all the features characteristic of autism. And the search continues.

One theoretical approach builds straight from the *cognitive style* exhibited by autistic persons on psychometric tests such as described in the last section. A common finding is that autistic persons perform at the superior range on tasks of visuospatial perception such as WISC Block Design, as well as other tests that require attention to the parts rather than the whole, such as the Embedded Figures Task (where one has to find hidden figures within a larger picture). On the basis of these findings, the psychologist Uta Frith and her colleagues (1989; Frith and Happé 1994) have proposed the *weak central coherence theory*, according to which autistic persons have a cognitive style that favors segmental (or local) over holistic (or global) information processing. According to this theory, a central deficit in autistic persons is their inability to integrate information from the environment into a meaningful whole. This theory explains the clinical observation that autistic persons notice the smallest change in their environment (such as when something is slightly moved from its usual place; Bosch 1962/1970; Kanner 1943). To some extent, it also explains the savant syndrome; that is, the isolated exceptional skills shown by many autistic persons in areas such as arts—most often drawing and music—and calculation, in spite of mental retardation (but see Mottron *et al.* 1999, for a different view).

However, experimental studies that specifically investigated autistic subjects' performance on tasks involving global and local processing yielded mixed results, depending on the context (e.g., the type or requirements of the tasks).[29] In addition, at least some of the differences may also be attributed to the wide range of abilities of those diagnosed as having one of the autism spectrum disorders. Contrary to the predictions of the central coherence theory, studies that specifically investigated subjects with Asperger syndrome did not find a significantly enhanced performance on tasks requiring local processing (Rodgers 2000), nor significantly impaired performance on tasks requiring global processing as compared to the control participants (Rinehart *et al.* 2000).

Other researchers studying autism have explored specific cognitive functions in autistic subjects, often positing a specific cognitive dysfunction as "the" core deficit in autism. For example, Michael Rutter (1978) has suggested that *language* dysfunctions may be the core deficit in autism. Language impairment is one of the defining features of autism (APA 1994) and about half of all autistic children never develop functional language (Bailey, Phillips, and Rutter 1996). Moreover, autistic children's parents typically report delay in language development as their first concern about the development of their children (Lord and Paul 1997).

Indeed, all aspects of language including features first described in clinical studies, such as echolalia, neologisms, pronoun reversal, and the language pragmatics (i.e., its social use) have been studied extensively in autistic subjects using a variety of tasks (for a recent review see Tager-Flusberg 2001b). The common finding of all these studies is that the pragmatic aspect of language is impaired. other aspects of language seem to be much more variable in autism.

For Asperger syndrome, it has been found that vocabulary and syntax are usually within the normal range of functioning, however, the pragmatic aspect of language remains seriously impaired (for a recent review see Twachtman Cullen 1998). Moreover, the speech patterns of subjects with Aspergers syndrome have been found to be more pedantic than that of high functioning autism subjects (Ghaziuddin 1996). with regard to the primacy of language deficit in autism, it is no longer considered among the most likely candidates for a core deficit. Moreover, it is currently believed that all language difficulties in people with autism stem from their lack of understanding intentionality (Tager-Flusberg 2001b).

Another psychological function that has been proposed as the core deficit in autism and which has been much researched is *attention* (Bryson, Wainwright-Sharp and Smith 1990; Burack *et al.* 1997). For example, Lovaas, Koegel and Schreibman (1979; also Burack 1994; Rincover and Ducharme 1987) found that the attention of autistic children is "overselective" (i.e., that they focus on a particular aspect of the environment and disregard the rest). However, it was also found that the attention of autistic persons can be "underselective," at least in the visual modality (Burack 1994). A similar pattern of inconsistent findings has been found with regard to another aspect of attention—the ability to shift attention. Although not all autistic persons are impaired on tasks of attentional shifting, at least some of them are, on at least some tasks (Allen and Courchesne 2001; Pascualvaca *et al.* 1998). Interestingly, some evidence suggests that, on some attentional shifting tasks, subjects with Asperger syndrome do not show the same impaired performance that individuals with high-functioning autism do (Rinehart *et al.* 2001). Finally, autistic children's ability for sustained attention does not seem to be impaired (Allen and Courchesne 2001).

Memory is another psychological function postulated as the main dysfunction in autism (Boucher and Warrington 1976; Rimland 1964). Although the most consistent research finding is that short- and long-term memory in autistic subjects is intact (Bennetto, Pennington and Rogers 1996), as is their ability to monitor the source of memories (Farrant, Blades and Boucher 1998). Some recent studies indicate that the processes and the strategies used by autistic subjects may be different than those used in other populations (Renner, Klinger and Klinger 2000; Toichi and Kamio 2002). One aspect of memory—*working memory* (i.e., capacity for holding and manipulating information relevant to the current task)—has received special attention in studies of autism; some studies have found that it is impaired in some autistic subjects (Bennetto *et al.* 1996); however, not all studies confirm this finding (Ozonoff and Strayer 2001).

Among the currently most popular theoretical accounts of autism is the *executive dysfunction hypothesis* of autism. (Executive function includes planning, inhibition of a pre-potent response, impulse control, problem-solving related to future goals, and flexibility of thought and action, among others; Ozonoff 1995; Ozonoff, Pennington and Rogers 1991; Pennington and Ozonoff 1996).[30] A common research finding is that autistic subjects have poor performance on some of the psychological tasks requiring executive functions, such as flexibility and planning, but not on tasks of inhibition (Hill 2004; Ozonoff and Jensen 1999). However, once again, the pattern of impairments varies across studies—and task requirements (see Liss *et al.* 2001; Russell, Jarrold and Hood 1999).[31] Although some researchers suggested that executive functions may be "uniquely impaired" in autistic persons (e.g., Ozonoff 1995, p.200), impairments in executive function have been found in many other disorders, including attention deficit hyperactivity disorder (ADHD), schizophrenia, Tourette syndrome, and obsessive-compulsive disorder (for recent reviews see Hill 2004 and Russell 1997). Interestingly, while Ozonoff, Pennington, and Rogers (1991) found that both subjects with Asperger syndrome and high functioning autism were impaired on executive function tasks, some more recent studies of executive function in subjects with Asperger syndrome did not find any impairment on the Wisconsin Card Sorting Test, a commonly used executive function task (Nyden *et al.* 1999). In a recent review, Baron-Cohen (2001) lists 20 such tasks.

Since impairments in social interaction and communication are defining characteristics of autism, it is no surprise that *social cognition* has been the main focus of many psychologists studying autism spectrum disorders. There have been numerous theoretical accounts that postulated different aspects of social cognition to be "the" core deficit in autism, and there have been hundreds of studies that tested these hypotheses.

The earliest studies of social cognition[32] focused on the ability of autistic children to understand emotions, form attachment relationships with their caregivers, and imitate others. These studies found that autistic children have great difficulty understanding their own and others' *emotions.* For example, autistic children find it hard to evaluate facial expressions (Hobson 1986; but see Ozonoff, Pennington and Rogers 1990, for contradicting results), name feelings (Hobson, Ouston and Lee 1989), understand what causes them (Baron-Cohen

1991), and empathize with others (Sigman *et al.* 1992; Yirmiya *et al.* 1992). They also find it hard to respond to affect in others and establish interpersonal relatedness (Hobson 1989, 1993).

However, contrary to initial reports about autistic children's *attachment* difficulties (Sigman and Mundy 1989; Sigman and Ungerer 1984), recent studies show that at least some autistic children develop normal secure attachment relations (Capps, Sigman and Mundy 1994; Rogers, Ozonoff and Maslin-Cole 1991). For example, children with high-functioning autism differentiate between their mothers and strangers and react differently to them. They also display other evidence of attachment, especially upon separation and reunion (Dissanayake and Sigman 2001). However, some studies suggest that the development of secure attachment may be delayed and its behavioral patterns altered (Rogers, Ozonoff and Maslin-Cole 1993).

Imitation skills too have been postulated as the core deficit in autism (Meltzoff and Gopnik 1993; Rogers and Pennington 1991). Both autistic children and adults have been found to have problems imitating simple motor actions and actions with objects (Charman *et al.* 1997; Rogers *et al.* 2003). However, as with previous functions, not all studies find that these skills are impaired in autistic persons (e.g., Hobson and Lee 1999; for a recent review, see Smith and Bryson 1994).

Currently the most popular among social cognition deficit hypotheses (and in fact, the most popular hypothesis among all) is the *Theory of Mind (ToM) deficit hypothesis* (Baron-Cohen, Leslie and Frith 1985). According to this view, the core deficit of autistic persons is their inability to attribute mental states (such as intentions, desires, and beliefs) to self and others (an ability known as Theory of Mind ability). Simon Baron-Cohen (1995), who, along with Alan Leslie and Uta Frith, was the first to use the Theory of Mind experimental paradigm with autistic children, has suggested that autistic persons are *mindblind*, that is, "blind to things like thought, beliefs, knowledge, desires, and intentions" (p.1). Similarly, for Uta Frith (1989), "To the autistic individual...mental states, such as [feeling,] knowing and believing, are...a mystery" (p.168). According to this theory, understanding oneself parallels understanding of others, and so these researchers claim that autistic individuals are also deficient in their ability to understand themselves, read their own minds, self-reflect, or produce self-reports (Baron-Cohen, *et al.* 1985, 1986; Baron-Cohen 1989a, b, c, 1995, 2001).

Research in this paradigm typically requires an understanding that others' beliefs will differ from one's own because that person was not privy to critical information. There are many different ToM tasks. The most popular ToM task used with autistic children is the Sally-Ann Task, a first-order false-belief task (Baron-Cohen *et al.* 1985). In this task the story with two main characters (dolls, Sally and Anne) is enacted: Sally hides a marble in a basket and then leaves the scene. During her absence, Anne moves the marble to a box. Children are asked where Sally will look for her marble when she comes back. Typically developing children are successful on first-order ToM tasks around four years of age, as are mentally retarded persons with a mental age of over four. However, only 20–25 per cent of autistic persons pass first-order ToM tasks at the typical age, although 38–60 per cent do eventually pass these tasks at a later age (Dahlgren and Trillingsgaard 1996).[33]

The ToM deficit hypothesis in autism has been criticized on many grounds: (1) it does not account for all the abnormal features of autism (particularly restricted interests and activities); (2) the deficit is not primary (i.e., the early symptoms are present quite before the ToM "emerges"); (3) the deficit is not specific to autism (i.e., it is found in deaf children (Peterson and Siegal 2000) and in persons with Down syndrome (Yirmiya *et al.* 1996; Zelazo *et al.* 1996)); and (4) at least some autistic persons can pass even high-order ToM tasks (Bowler 1992; Ozonoff, Rogers and Pennington 1991). Moreover, some of the posited deficits in autistic persons were not found when "looked for"; for example, difficulties reporting intentions when they are different from the outcome, monitoring of goal-directed actions, monitoring basic actions (Russell and Hill 2001), or understanding emotions (Rieffe, Meerum Terwogt and Stockmann 2000) (for a recent critical review of the Theory of Mind hypothesis of autism see also Tager-Flusberg 2001a).[34]

Finally, some experts have postulated that the primary deficit in autism is the inability of autistic infants to share their experience and attention with others—a capacity known as *joint attention* (Sigman and Mundy 1989). This capacity develops at the end of the first year of life and allows infants to look in the direction in which another person is looking and to follow a pointing gesture. There have been several independent studies that confirm a specific developmental deficit, or delay, in joint attention in autistic children (Baron-Cohen *et al.* 1996; Leekam, Lopez and Moore 2000; Lord 1995; Loveland and Landry 1986; Mundy, Sigman and Kasari 1990; Osterling and Dawson 1994). Since joint attention is a complex mental function that combines attentional, motivational, emotional and cognitive elements, and since it emerges relatively early in development, it holds particular promise for early identification of autism and its understanding as a *developmental* disorder.[35]

Reflections

All these different approaches have provided some potentially useful information. However, as to their main goal—finding a cognitive function that can explain the behavior of autistic persons—they have failed, as none of the functions studied, considered alone, has this much explanatory power. Perhaps Hans Asperger's reaction to cognitive deficit hypotheses of his time is worth repeating here:

> the child cannot understand mime, gesture or facial expression and cannot react to it. But this seems too simple in my opinion. When such a child *wants* to, is able to want to understand the demands of the environment and the world around him, then he understands them very well indeed! The fault is more central though not in any single function. It is the inability to attend or take an interest. After all "interest" means, in English, "is among" and in German, "to be among" and this is just what they are not able to be. (1979, p.50, emphasis original)

In our next section, we consider how some of this discussion bears on Teodor and his self-understanding.

Self-understanding: The developmental perspective

A few studies have specifically addressed development of *self-awareness* in autistic children. They investigated self-recognition (Dawson and McKissick 1984), development of self-concept (Lee and Hobson 1998), self-perception (Capps, Sigman and Yirmiya 1995), and self-monitoring in autistic children and adolescents (Hill and Russell 2002; Russell and Hill 2001). Since this book specifically examines Teodor's self-understanding, we will consider the main findings about self-understanding of autistic children in some detail.

In the first study to specifically explore self-understanding of autistic children and adolescents (aged 9 years and 3 months–16 years and 10 months), Lisa Capps and her colleagues (1995) found that, as compared to non-autistic children matched on mental age, autistic subjects have lower estimations of their overall self-worth and think of themselves as less competent in the social and physical, but not the cognitive/scholastic, domains. In another study, of autistic children and adolescents aged 9–19, Anthony Lee and Peter Hobson (1998) found that autistic subjects' understanding of themselves differed significantly from that of subjects matched on mental age, but only in the number and quality of *social* self-statements. They also differed in the quality—but not the number—of self-statements for physical, active, and psychological aspects of self.

TEODOR'S SELF-PERCEPTION PROFILE FOR CHILDREN

Our first tool for assessing Teodor's self-understanding was Susan Harter's (1985) Self-Perception Profile for Children, a psychological instrument specifically designed to measure children's self-concept through their evaluations in one general (global self-worth) and five specific areas: (1) scholastic competence; (2) social acceptance; (3) athletic competence; (4) physical appearance; and (5) behavioral conduct.[36] This instrument has two parallel forms, one for adults who know the child well, and one for the child. We begin by considering how adults who know Teodor well evaluated him in five specific domains using this formal evaluation instrument (the adult form does not include a global evaluation domain).[37]

Three individuals, Teodor's mother, father, and Teodor's former teaching assistant (TA), filled out a rating scale of the child's actual behavior.[38] The three adult raters find Teodor very good looking and gave the highest rating to his physical appearance (mean score 4)[39] and the lowest score to his social acceptance (mean of about 1.5). They agreed within half a point on their evaluations of Teodor's performance in athletic competence and behavioral conduct domains, with scores between 2 and 3 in these domains.

However, for scholastic competence there was more discrepancy. One way to account for this discrepancy is that the raters all know Teodor in different scholastic contexts, and may be using different criteria to judge his competence. Teodor's father helps him with math and science, mother with social science studies and language arts, and the TA with in-class assignments in all areas. We already know that Teodor's father thinks Teodor is doing much better in math and science than his report card indicates. He may be judging Teodor's potential ability regardless of his performance on school tests. The mother's assessment is perhaps based on actual success on his report card and from her experience with helping Teodor with social science studies and language arts. The fact that the teaching assistant's mean score for this domain fell between the father's and the mother's supports this interpretation since he assists Teodor in all domains and knows both Teodor's actual performance and potential scholastic abilities.

Teodor gave himself relatively low scores on all subscales of this instrument (his highest score—2.50 on the physical appearance subscale—is still half a point lower than the mean of the sixth grade boys in Harter's study—3.01). In fact, the Self-Perception Profile for Children Teodor generated suggests he is barely competent in all six domains. More specifically, according to his self-evaluations, Teodor believes that he is somewhat competent in four domains (physical appearance (2.50), athletic competence and social acceptance (both 2.17), and scholastic competence (2.00)); and somewhat incompetent in two domains, behavioral conduct and global self-worth (both 1.67).[40] (A profile of Teodor's scores on Harter's scale and how it compares to the ratings of the individuals' who know him , as well as to the scores obtained by Grade 6 boys in Harter's study (1985) is presented in Table 4.1.)

Table 4.1: Self-perception scores for Teodor and for grade-six boys in Harter's study (1985)

Subscale	*Teodor*	*Grade six boys*	*Mother*	*Father*	*TA*
Physical appearance	2.50	3.01	4.00	4.00	4.00
Athletic competence	2.17	3.08	2.00	2.00	1.60
Social acceptance	2.17	3.00	1.60	1.30	1.30
Scholastic competence	2.00	3.01	2.30	3.30	2.60
Behavioral conduct	1.67	2.85	3.00	2.60	3.00
Global self-worth	1.67	3.12			

Reflections

But is this profile accurate? From the adults' perspectives, Teodor underestimates his competences in three domains, and overestimates them in two. For physical appearance, his mean score of 2.5 ("somewhat nice looking") was well below that of adults, who gave him a mean score of 4.0 ("really good looking"), the highest possible score. Similarly, Teodor's rating of his competence in domains of behavioral conduct and scholastic competences (scores of 1.67 and 2.00 respectively) seem somewhat low relative to all the adults' ratings (scores from 2.60 to 3.00 on the behavioral conduct subscale and from 2.30 to 3.30 on the scholastic competence subscale). On the other hand, Teodor's ratings in the domains of social and athletic competences (scores of 2.17 in both domains) were somewhat high relative to the adult ratings (whose scores ranged from 1.60 to 2.00 on the athletic competence subscale, and from 1.3 to 1.60 on the social acceptance subscale). How to explain these differences? One way to find out is to ask Teodor to explain his answers.

A CLINICAL INTERVIEW

To gain a better understanding of Teodor's self-evaluations on the Self-Perception Profile for Children, we conducted an in-depth clinical interview with him, in which we asked him to explain why he answered as he did for half (18) of his answers on this questionnaire. (The questions were chosen to probe the greatest diversity of Teodor's responses within each domain.)[41]

Physical appearance

According to Teodor's overall score of his physical appearance (2.50), one would expect Teodor to be generally pleased by his looks. And he is. When asked why he circled that it is "sort of true" that he is good looking,[42] he said, "I kind of look nice." However, Teodor's scores in the physical domain range from 1 to 4. One wonders what aspects of his physical appearance deserved such drastically different evaluations. An analysis of three of Teodor's responses related to this aspect of the self revealed the following: Teodor is really happy with some aspects of his physical appearance (his height and weight)[43] but very unhappy with the others (his pimples, and how his looks change when crying)—so much so that he wishes his physical appearance were different.[44]

Teodor observed that when he cries his looks change in a way that he does not like; he said, "[W]hen I cry, I'm not quite good looking." He also said that he used to cry a lot and that his father "barely ever cries," adding, "I wanna be like a real man." When asked how he knows that his face does not look nice when he cries, he replied, "I can *feel* it." When asked where, he said: "I feel my face moving, and my mouth and my eyes and the tears coming, and the sound." This explanation suggests that one source of Teodor's negative self-evaluations about his physical appearance is his kinesthetic perception (i.e., the *feeling* of tensing of his facial muscles when he cries).

However, the main source of Teodor's dissatisfaction with his body seems to be his pimples; they came up as an issue when he was asked to elaborate on three answers about his physical self-concept.[45] Thus, when asked why he chose to answer that he really "wishes his body were different," rather than that he is "happy with his body the way it is,"[46] he said, "because I have lots of—things like that—pimples...and I don't like that." Ljiljana counted five pimples on his cheeks and his forehead. When asked whether he thought that five pimples are a lot, he replied, "No, but they *feel* ugly," and mentioned the sensation he feels when he touches his skin.[47] When asked why he does not like the way he looks with pimples, he repeated that it is how he "*feel*[*s*] them—they are just ugly." When asked whether he heard from somebody that he or his pimples are ugly, he said no. So the other source of Teodor's negative evaluations of his body seems to be his tactile perception (we return to this issue in the next chapter).

Athletic competence

Teodor feels that when it comes to sports, he is somewhat competent (2.17). When asked why he wishes that he "could be a lot better at sports,"[48] he answered, "I'd be so smart." When asked why he answered that he is not very good at sports,[49] he provided the following explanation:

> At my sports sometimes—I can't pay attention—or sometimes when my friend asks me, "Do you wanna play with the ball?" I say no, but since he moved and I don't get to see him always, I don't do that anymore. Plus sometimes—I don't—I just can't do well.

And this is how Teodor explains what not paying attention in sports means:

> Like when I play tennis—sometimes when the ball was going to the left, like, I'm here and the ball was going there [shows] to the left, I couldn't see it. I mean—I mean I saw it, but when it went to the left, I didn't run—I just stayed. Victor said, "You just stay and if it comes to you, you throw it. If it doesn't, you don't." Victor said that, but that's not true. Sometimes I do that.

In addition to having difficulties with attention in sports, Teodor believes that he has difficulties with sports rules, which he calls "additional rules." He said, "*The Life* [the board game] with no additional rules—it's easy." But in sports, "some rules are hard." For example, soccer has "the specific rules [which] are always or almost always different." He said that soccer would be easy "if there [were] no additional rules." Basketball too has too many rules and he "can't remember all of them." In other words, for Teodor, games have only one rule. Basketball has the rule of trying to put the ball into the basket; all other rules of the game are "additional rules" that make it hard. Surprisingly, he also said that he "could do well at just about any new sports or activity he hasn't tried before,"[50] and added, "I just have to pay attention to the rules."

Teodor also believes that he cannot run as fast as other children: " They can run very fast—um—and I can't—*that* fast." However, he believes that he is good at running "approximately two" laps.

Social acceptance

Teodor's subscores on this subscale range from 1 to 3 (mean score of 2.17). When asked to elaborate on his answers pertaining to his social competences, Teodor expressed a wish to have: (a) "more friends," (b) "new friends", and (c) girl friends.

(a) Even though Teodor feels that he has a lot of friends[51] (i.e., "more than four"),[52] he also wishes to have a lot *more*.[53] He observed that some other children have more friends, "In my class there is one person who has six or even more friends." From this, Teodor concluded that he, too, should have more friends, and when asked whether he belongs to a group of children who "would like to have alot [sic] more friends," or to a group who has "as many friends as they want,"[54] he chose the first description and circled "really true for me" (a score of 1.0). He explained, "I don't have as many friends as other people have."

(b) Teodor also "wishes" to have "*new friends*," but could not explain why, besides saying that some children just never played with him.

(c) Finally, Teodor also wishes he had more friends "that are *girls* [because] the girls that I like don't tease me." (We will have more to say about this a little later, after we discuss the other aspects of Teodor's self-evaluation.)

Scholastic competence

According to the score he obtained on the scholastic competence subscale (a score of 2.0), Teodor does not consider himself to be very competent scholastically, for three reasons. First, he cannot concentrate on schoolwork as much as he should, "Sometimes I don't know what to do because I look at pictures,[55] and it's hard for me to pay attention." This happens even when he is doing easy math questions such as adding, and so he does not "pay attention and forget[s] to carry the one." Second are the bad marks on the tests that he sometimes gets—in spite of studying, "Sometimes, I get, like, poor marks on tests. Like in grade four, I studied for a test and I got 'R.' So, like that—I'm not good." Third, Teodor might have found a discrepancy when comparing his knowledge of school subjects and about public transit to that of other children, "I am smart at the TTC" and "kids my age are smart usually at math and at language arts, not at TTC."[56] However, Teodor does consider himself to be "smart at math" and "good at making poems about [him]self."[57]

But, above all, Teodor views himself as "smart at TTC." During the interview, Teodor often spoke about his "smartness" and his knowledge about public transit. He said, "I studied lots and lots of TTC maps, or routes—how they go—and they made me smart." Teodor also contrasted his interest in public transit to that in school subjects. He said that even though he hates to read school stuff, he likes to read TTC stuff and stories that he writes about his trips. In fact, during the introductory part of the Self-Perception Profile for Children, Teodor demonstrated that he learned a great deal from reading "TTC stuff." When told that he will be filling out the survey, Teodor said:

> I know the word "survey" from TTC...from an update when it said that they are going to put new train cars on trains, like, more—it was a survey. Like, about "How do you feel about more train cars?" "How would you like the tables to be in the new ones [as opposed to] the old ones"...but I didn't do it, I just kept it [the brochure].

Behavioral conduct

Teodor scored 1.67 in this domain. When asked why he circled that it is sort of true that he often does not do "the right thing,"[58] Teodor listed four "wrong" things he does: cheat, argue, make fun of people, and hurt their feelings. With regard to cheating, he said:

> Sometimes, like, not lots of times, but very little, very little, once in a while... I make sure no one sees me and I cheat... Like, at one test I got B because I cheated... Like, my notes—I knew where they were, and I made sure no teachers were looking around and—I looked, and—then I—pulled the paper so I put it in slowly so that—the—the teachers don't hear "BOOM!" for the papers moving. Like, a few times.

Interestingly, Teodor said that he cheated in spite of knowing that it is not the right thing to do, but the temptation was too great, "I *wanted* to, because I wanna get a good mark... Because if I get a good mark, I can go with TTC."

Teodor also said, "Sometimes I argue," and gave the following example:

> Sometimes I have to—sometimes I have—like, my mother says—like, she told me to read when I am home, and—I mean, not when I am home, anytime in the day, and I chose to read when I usually read with her, and—but not usually, and when it's late, she said, "No, we are not reading, it's too late." Then I said, "FINE! You told me—to read every day, well, reading today—CANCELLED!"

Teodor also said, "Sometimes I make fun of people":

> Like a boy whose name is Sam in my class—not this one that lives beside me, another one—his last name is Kort, with a K at the beginning, and—if he says that I am annoying, like that, and *he know that, and I know that too, for some people I am annoying,*[59] um, I said, "Mr. Kort!", and then, he was saying, like, something that meant, WOULD YOU STOP IT, in a voice like—like that, because, like, some teachers like—a boy whose name is Albert, and his last name is Bard, the teacher wasn't saying, "Albert!" when he wasn't doing something well, sometimes he was saying, "Mr. Bard." And I take that information to *make fun of other people's names.*

Finally, Teodor said, "Sometimes when I behave bad, I hurt my mother's feelings... And my grandmother's:"

> Like, when I blow like that [blows], I don't mean to blow right in her face... And—she said, "One more time you do it, and I'm not gonna talk to you." But I forgot. She gave me a chance. But, like, *I like when I blow* [blows] *and in one second the hairs flies up*—I like that. Like if I blow [blows] then—and she does [shows how she moves her head backwards and makes a face] like that in her face, like, I blow in her eyes, or in her nose—I don't mean to do that—*the main thing I mean* is like to blow the hair [blows], and then the hair [shows hair going up] flies up a little bit—like that.

When asked why he answered that he "often find[s] it hard to behave,"[60] Teodor explains:

> Sometimes, if my mother doesn't like something, but the other people I visit like it, I keep on doing it... Like I said with some people, a word... And, like, my mother was doing that [makes a serious face], which means she was saying, "Hey," so she was telling me, um—[meaning: that's not a proper word to use] but, like, um, the people I visited, like—they laugh at that word. And laughing means, they like it.

Global self-worth

A clinical interview shows that two main sources for Teodor's judgment about his global self-worth (score 1.67) are the way he behaves and the things he does not know. He circled that he really doesn't like "the way [he is] leading [his] life"[61] and the reason he gives is "because, like, I don't know lots of things—I know TTC—as—as I know TTC now I *should* know things about life." Things about life, for Teodor, are "math, language arts, everything I know." Teodor remembers what his mother said: "My mother said, 'When are you gonna have those pictures away and learn new stuff?' and she said, 'I thought next year there will be less TTC.'"

Reflections

We begin this section by exploring two questions. First, how do we interpret the discrepancy between Teodor's evaluations of himself and those of others obtained using this instrument. And second, does Teodor really think that he is as incompetent as his self-portrait on the Self-Perception Profile for Children suggests?

First, when Teodor's ratings of his competences are compared to those of individuals who know him well, we find they are very different. However, when we look at Teodor's explanations, his reasoning behind them is more or less adequate: he considers relevant information and makes appropriate judgments, but in ways that are not immediately apparent—sometimes because he uses information only accessible to him. Most often, Teodor places a different importance on the information he considers to evaluate his competences.

For example, in evaluating his *physical appearance*, Teodor mostly used tactile and kinesthetic information. These are relevant sources of information; however, most people judge their physical appearance based on how they look, and this is what was considered in evaluations of Teodor we obtained from others. This discrepancy in kinds of information considered contributed to the differences between Teodor's and others' judgments of his physical appearance. Another important factor that might have played a role in Teodor's lower estimates of his physical appearance than those of others is that Teodor comes from a family in which there are cultural norms about reporting self-evaluations about one's appearance according to which openly expressed high self-evaluations are not encouraged (see Hagger *et al.* 2003; Markus and Kitayama 1991).

In the domain of *athletic competence*, Teodor identified paying attention, knowing rules of sports, and being fast, as relevant to his self-evaluation. Teodor believes that he is not particularly good at sports because he is not very good at these aspects of sports, and in particular with complex rules he finds hard to learn. He called these rules "additional," implying that there is more to the sports than the basic rules, which seem to be just out of his grasp. Moreover, sometimes he feels that there are too many rules. However, Teodor also believes that he *could* excel in sports if he just paid more attention to these additional sport rules. So perhaps this optimistic approach to his competences could account for a slight discrepancy between his and adult raters' evaluations in this domain.

In the *social competence* domain, Teodor was asked to compare himself to other children in regard to the number of friends he has, and he did. The comparisons he made are adequate. However, here too, there is a sense of optimism regarding having more and new friends. Teodor feels that he could have more friends, if he finds ones willing to play his games. We will return to this point later in the chapter.

Although most of his report card marks are good, Teodor's assessment of his *scholastic competence* refers to cases when he got a bad mark, in spite of studying. So Teodor may not be taking his marks at face value, but rather considers the effort he has to put into studying to get them, which seems valid. For example, Teodor considers how hard it is for him to focus on school tasks when public transit pictures just keep popping up in his mind—and he knows this better than anybody else. Finally, when he considers the difference between his scholastic and his public transit knowledge, he is entirely correct that his knowledge of the TTC is much greater than is his knowledge of any school subject.[62]

As for his *behavioral conduct*, Teodor knows, and almost always follows, the rules of proper behavior. He knows that cheating, arguing and hurting others' feelings are not proper things to do, and he believes that anyone who does these kinds of things (as he sometimes does) cannot be said to behave properly. In this, Teodor reasons just like other children his age. The only factor Teodor does not take into account (as adults do) is how often he does these inappropriate things—and the truth is, not very often. And what he considers to be hurting others' feelings probably does not seem so bad to them. True, Teodor's parents may convey their dissatisfaction with Teodor's misbehavior to him, but they certainly do not believe it to be that bad.

The clinical interview shows that Teodor's *global self-worth* estimations are based on two "domains:" his behavior, and his knowledge about life. Thus, he said that his behavior is not good, and therefore the way he is leading his life is not good. We also heard him say that his mother said that he should know about life as much as he knows about public transit. Therefore, it is possible that he identified knowing about different aspects of life with living it. However, it does not seem to us that these two domains are what he considers important. He clearly indicated that this is what others deem important. Had Teodor been asked about his self-worth *after* he talked about his competences in public transit, his estimations might have been quite different. That is, since he was asked *only* about domains in which he is not very interested, and, thus, perhaps not very competent, this might have led him to think of his behavior in these domains, and not in a domain he deems important, when asked global self-worth questions. This interpretation is supported by all accounts by persons who know him; as Teodor's mother said, Teodor "feels good, and the world for him is good."

Second, is it true that Teodor does not feel good about himself? The in-depth interview gives us a first glimpse into Teodor's inner world. We now hear him speak in his own voice and we get to know him a lot better than we do from the answers on a forced-choice, paper and pencil questionnaire. When explaining the choices he made on the questionnaire, Teodor did not seem to be concerned with any measured aspects of his competences, nor to have a low self-esteem—which his score of 1.67 on global self-worth suggests. To the contrary, Teodor seems very proud, not only of his TTC knowledge, but also of the general knowledge he has acquired through "studying TTC."

Teodor is extremely optimistic even for domains in which he sees a difference between himself and other children (e.g., in the athletic, social, or scholastic domains). Even in the physical domain, in which he wished his body were different, his explanation did not convey the sense of any really big dissatisfaction with his body—rather, he just wished he did not have pimples.

Therefore, for Teodor, the Self-Perception Profile for Children was not a very valid instrument for capturing his self-perceptions; open-ended questions seem like a better way to know his real feelings about himself.

We believe that the above discussion clearly suggests that for children with Asperger syndrome, self-concept questionnaires need to incorporate questions about their domain of main interest. Teodor deeply values his TTC knowledge, which is not the case for knowledge he has acquired in school, where he only wants to get a good mark because he will be rewarded with a trip. He even cheats on the tests, sometimes, to be sure his mark will be good enough to merit a trip.

As mentioned earlier, a research study by Lisa Capps and her colleagues (1995) found that autistic children have lower estimations of their overall self-worth and think of themselves as less competent in two domains, social and physical. When we administered the Self-Perception Profile for Children (although not the same version[63] used in this other study) to Teodor, we found both similarities and differences. First, Teodor's performance indicated that he too has lower estimations of his overall self-worth. Second, the two domains reported to be the most deficient in the study by Lisa Capps and her colleagues, physical appearance and social acceptance, were not so in Teodor's case; on the contrary, they were ranked the highest by him. Third, Teodor's scholastic competence score was low, which was not the case in the study by Lisa Capps and her colleagues.

But, as William James (1890) and more recently Susan Harter suggest, global self-worth is "determined, in part, by how competent or adequate one is in those domains deemed important" (Harter 1985, p.18). The fact that Teodor was not asked about the domain of his *highest* competencies is reflected in his low estimations on the global self-worth subscale. Teodor considers his competence in public transit as most important to him, as seen from Teodor's interview and in previous accounts by others. Thus, Teodor's low estimations of his global self-worth are an artifact of the questionnaire, not a true estimation of how Teodor really feels about himself.

What else do we learn about Teodor from this clinical interview? Teodor's elaborations of his answers about social acceptance on the Harter's questionnaire go beyond issues of his popularity and the number of friends he wishes to have (the main aspects of social competences measured by this instrument), and provide a window into his social life and his reasoning about it. In this section, we consider two more aspects of his "social self": first, how he plays with other children and second, his social reasoning, or more specifically, how he understands friendship.

First, when Teodor plays with children, they almost always play "his bus and train games," under *his* conditions. First, children can join his game only at particular places, "[Kevin] can come into my bus when I stop somewhere." Second, they can follow him, "[I]f I'm playing bus and Kevin, like, follows me, that's okay." And third, he cannot stop his game and begin a new one when a friend comes—he has to finish his game first (or, in his words, "I ha[ve] to—continue *my* route.").[64]

As he explains:

> I have to get back to the terminal at my house, or—at least to the first terminal I stop at—like—let's say—I'm—I stopped somewhere, but that's not my final destination—I continue and, at my final destination, I say, "Out of service," and then I go to my house—and I am out of service—I am not in service to carry people—um—I go to my house—I put the bus [a bicycle] there and I play [with a friend].

On rare occasions, he can "finish" the game a bit faster, when others are calling him: "[S]ometimes I can, like, pretend that a new driver was waiting for me, but I don't always like that."

In addition, Teodor does not like to be *invited* to play—he wants to be the one who invites: "I don't like when he [Kevin] comes and asks me to come out. I like if he plays with me—if I come out—without anyone calling me—and then he starts playing with me. I like that more." Moreover, he refers to his friends' invitations to play as something that "disturbs" him. He said:

Teodor:	With Kevin—like—I do play but he always disturbs me, and he—and he knows that and on purpose wants that.
Ljiljana:	How does he disturb you?
Teodor:	He comes, he sees the sign [on his door that says that he is busy; Figure 4.4] but—he simply wants me to play—
Ljiljana:	So he disturbs you by asking you to come and play?
Teodor:	Yeah.

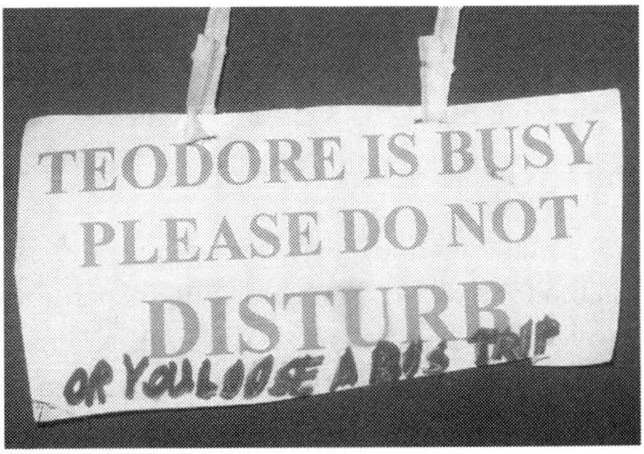

Figure 4.4: Teodor's house-door sign

Teodor's games also have to be played according to the time schedule, and if a friend comes and "disturbs" this schedule, he does not like that. Here is his description of an "incident" with Victor:

> And Victor one day was talking to me along my way—when I didn't realize that traffic was stopped—I was thirty minutes late, and I had to call them to tell them. [Ljiljana: Call whom?] The employees, to tell them that I am late.[65]... And like—Victor talks to me—I say, "Wait a minute, CAN'T YOU SEE I AM TALKING ON THE PHONE?!" [yells] and then I talk.[66]

In school, too, Teodor finds friends' invitations to play, or talk, disturbing.

Ljiljana:	Why would you like more [friends]?
Teodor:	Because, like, at recess, like, I can just draw—not lots of people wanna play with me.
Ljiljana:	Why not?
Teodor:	Because—some people do, but, like, I played with them a lot and now I wanna draw.
Ljiljana:	Uh-huh, but why did you say that not a lot of people want to play with you?
Teodor:	Because, like, some people have many people who they talk to in class—when they shouldn't, and at recess they all have fun.
Ljiljana:	Oh. So, they play together then at recess.
Teodor:	Uh-huh, but, like, some people this year—that just passed, um—in the other door—lots of people in my class plus some people in the other class, all played baseball, like, more than ten.
Ljiljana:	Uh-huh, at recess?
Teodor:	Uh-huh.
Ljiljana:	Uh-huh. And?
Teodor:	And Kevin—no—some people talk to me, like, when they want to ask me a question, um, like, if I have tape—because they need some tape—but, like, Kevin wants to talk to me, but I don't wanna talk to him because, like, in the class, I shouldn't talk.
Ljiljana:	But what about recess—let's talk about recess.
Teodor:	He keeps on wanting to play with me, and I can't do what I want.

Second, Teodor's understanding of friendship is unique. This can be illustrated in three related issues: Teodor's way of friend-making; his criteria for considering somebody a friend (or not); and his ways of dealing with friends' "bad behavior."

First, Teodor believes that it is not particularly hard to make friends. He explains:

> I could easily go to a boy or to a girl, and ask him or her, "Do you wanna play with me?" and I could play with that person every day and—um—and then I could ask him or her the phone number and invite him or her over to my house to play, and then we could be friends.

However, he says that although "I know how I can do it...I don't do it most of the time." But he used this strategy once, with a girl: "When I was in grade four...I met her in a park and asked her if she wants to play with me... And I became friends with her... But she moved to the US."

Second, when Teodor was asked about why he considers some children to be his friends, he offers different criteria for different children. For example, he considers Kevin to be his friend because "he's playing with me, he's, like, bringing me transfers, and he's behaving good." Also, "He brings me cars to play with, and...[h]e, like, makes jokes with me." Victor is a friend because he is "playing with me like that." Charlie is a friend because "we just have fun together." Jay is a friend because "he is helping me to wash desks, because sometimes I have to leave some rooms not washed, like, the bell rings and, like, two or three rooms—I can't wash desks in them, I mean classes—and he washes—I wash some desks and he washes more...or he washes one room and I wash the other one, so we can finish faster." And Alicia is a friend because she too helps with cleaning the desks. Harry, however, is a friend for yet another reason:

> Because, like, before he was talking to me, and [I] said, "Do you wanna come to my birthday?" and he said, "Yes" but he couldn't, because he had to do something, and he said, "Are you my friend?" and whenever someone says that, I say okay, but if later on they are my friend and they behave bad, I try my best not to stop.

When asked whether he considers a friend anybody who asks him "Are you my friend?" he answered, yes, if "they are not bad people." And he made a clear distinction between "bad people" and "bad behavior."[67] Thus, children who always do things to him that he does not like are "bad people," but children who play (or help) him are his friends, and when they do things he does not like, they are "just behaving bad." Teodor said:

> In the [school] bus when someone fights with me, that person is bad[68]...[or] people who laugh at me,[69] but, like, if they are not bad people—if I don't consider them bad when they do that—if before they weren't bad people—I just say their behavior is bad, I just say that. Like if Kevin behaves bad, like, if he rips my paper when I draw...I'm not saying, "You're a bad boy; you're not my friend," I don't say that. I say that he has bad behavior.

However, even the children he considers "bad people" can become Teodor's friends, once they start behaving the way he likes. In fact, two of his current friends used to be "bad people": Charlie, the boy who was fighting with him for the first seat in the bus "was [first] blocking my way...in front of me and [now] I do it back, and he likes that. And, like, we just have fun together;" and Jay (who now helps him with the desks) "before—when I was going up the slide, he was pulling me down—always."

Third, when one of Teodor's friends "behaves bad," Teodor has a special way of teaching him to be a "better friend":

> I have a book with a consequence schedule (Figure 4.5), and—oh—if you do that, what do I do, and at the top [shows in the air] it says what he does, and it says "Kevin," "Victor," and in that square over there [points in the air]—it's not quite a square—it's like a rectangle—I write the consequences. Like, if I say, "Annoying so much," and then, "Victor," it says, "Next TTC trip cancelled"—he doesn't come with me on the next trip... I write "Trips cancelled"—like him coming—not that I don't go. "Kevin," "Victor," and I do one line and that means one, if I do five, it means five trips cancelled. And, like, saying, "None of your business," "Victor—one," so now I get to say it to him...like, I show him, "See, you have that much trips cancelled, now I'm adding one more" if I have to—I show him.

Teodor has a "consequence schedule" only for two of his best friends, Kevin and Victor, who like to go with him on his trips.[70] He explains:

> [Harry, another friend] doesn't ask, "If you go on a TTC trip, can I come with you?" He doesn't—he barely asks that, but if he starts behaving bad and he wants to play with me, I take away privileges, and I have to add one more person [in the consequence book]. But other people don't have consequences.

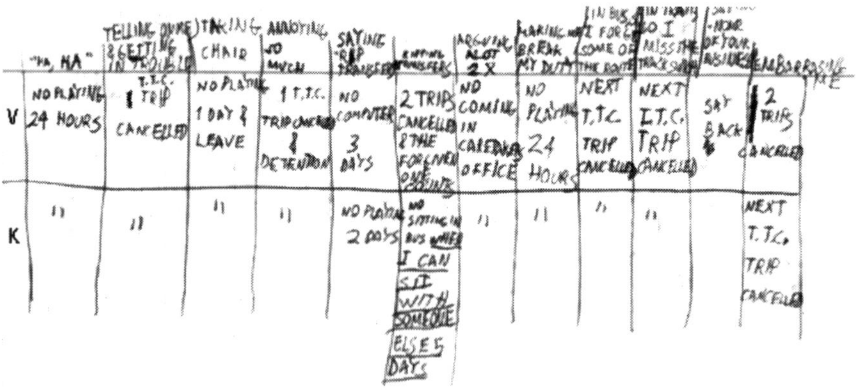

Figure 4.5: Teodor's "consequence schedule"

Here are two examples of what counts as bad behavior that deserves the "trip-cancelled" consequence. For example, in school, "In the caretaker's office, Kevin and Victor, if I get up off a chair and they take it and don't give it back, they have a consequence." At home, Teodor made a sign that he put on his house door on which he wrote "Teodor IS BUSY; PLEASE DO NOT DISTURB; OR YOU LOOSE A BUS TRIP" (Figure 4.4). He explained that this is for his friends when they come to ask him to come and play.

Even though Teodor uses the "trip-cancelled" consequence the most often, he also uses the same consequences that his friends use with him:

> [Victor] was saying when I embarrass him, like I say—let's say I say, "You little," and then someone looks at him—I embarrass him and he doesn't sit with me on the [school] bus one day. Because of that I said when he rip my transfer—did I tell you—he ripped it once and then I cried, "No, give it back," I had to yell, and he did. No, he didn't take it—he gave me three and the other one he kept and ripped—only once—and I taped it back, and he made me cry. And, like, I said, "Because of that I'm not sitting with you" or "talking to you one week," or no—I think just "playing with you"—I mean no—"sitting with you in the bus."

Finally, Teodor has some consequences that he uses as a means of taking care of his friends. He explains:

> I tell on him [Kevin] lots of times... Sometimes I need too, to take care of him. [For example, when] the teacher said, "If you don't stay in, you have a detention—if your name is on the board"—for recess at lunch, and Kevin has to help and his name is on the board. And I needed to tell...his father in order to make him not get a detention and he did stay in. So that's a good thing to tell.

However, when somebody else does the same to him, Teodor does not consider it as "taking care" of him, and instead counts it as bad behavior, which deserves the worst consequence (i.e., "next TTC trip cancelled") (see Figure 4.5, the first row). Similarly, when other children (who do not "have consequences"), try to "take care" of him, Teodor feels that they have bad intentions. Thus, he said of a boy in his classroom, "Sometimes when he wants to be bad, like, um, he wants to be mean to me, he says it loud when I draw—he says, 'Teodor man, stop playing with your stuff!'—loud so that the teacher hears it."

In sum, there are other things we learned about Teodor from the clinical interview beyond what Harter's instrument specifically targeted in terms of self-perception. The most salient seem to be about Teodor's interaction with other children. Thus, we learned that, while wishing to have more new friends, Teodor is actually avoiding the friends he has (and that he finds their invitations to play "disturbing"). And although Teodor says he wants to play with others, he wants to do or play what he wishes. Teodor also knows that not many children want to play with him. We learned, too, about Teodor's understanding of friendship. He believes that a friend is one who plays and jokes with you, and who helps you. Teodor says he knows "how to" make friends, but does not do so very often. Finally, we learned that Teodor has a special way to "help" his friends when they sometimes misbehave (by "giving them consequences" and telling to the teacher), but he does not like it when they tell on him.

Though it was not the purpose of this study to explore Teodor's understanding of others' minds, given what he said in this clinical interview and other accounts of him, in at least two instances, Teodor comments seem to contradict predictions of the Theory of Mind's hypothesis of autism that he would not be able to understand another's point of view. For example, although autistic persons are supposedly incapable of deceiving (Russell *et al.* 1991), Teodor successfully cheated on a test. He was able to trick the teacher by paying attention to information from different sources simultaneously and adjusting his actions accordingly. So not only does Teodor understand that there are different ways others can discover his wrongdoing (e.g., by hearing or seeing him), he can also apply this knowledge when it is important to him. This observation is consistent with a study that found that children understand others' minds better when they need to (Chandler, Fritz and Hala 1989).[71] But certainly the best example is when Teodor spoke about how he is distinct from others in the Damon and Hart Self-Understanding Interview. By saying that a person in Bucharest would not know and could not know about bus routes in Canada because they have not had the experience of them, while he knows them because he has had the necessary experience, he addresses all the critical features of a first-order Theory of Mind task. In fact, by saying that he knows that his parents test him and continue to test him until he can demonstrate what he knows, one is tempted to think he has some understanding of second-order Theory of Mind (that he knows that they know what he does or does not know). Of course, once again, he may demonstrate this only in situations such as this, in which he is deeply interested and motivated to understand others' perspectives. Indeed, this is what Hans Asperger (1944/1991, p.73) observed in the day-to-day lives of autistic children he took care of.

Teodor also showed empathy in a number of situations reported by him and by his family members. He both understands and is empathetic (emotionally responsive) to the feelings of others, especially to their distress. He also takes care of friends who are hurt, and of his grandmother when they go on trips. Teodor's empathic reactions towards people he knows stand in sharp contrast to most findings from experimental studies. For example, Marian Sigman and her colleagues (1992) found that autistic children are less responsive to other people's distress than are comparison groups. Autistic children paid less attention and showed less reaction to the pretended distress of their mothers than did comparison groups of typically developing and mentally retarded children. Bacon *et al.* (1998), using simulated distress by an unfamiliar adult, found little empathy in autistic children. Yirmiya *et al.* (1992) also found little understanding and empathy in their high-functioning autistic children when they viewed videotaped events intended to elicit empathy. However, in one recent study by James Blair (1999), autistic children showed appropriate responses, as recorded via electrodermal responses to slides with distress cues (e.g., crying). Although his study concerns only autonomic response to distress of others, and not children's emotional experience, Blair believes that autistic children may be "capable of experiencing an emotion having witnessed the distress cues of others" (p.483).

TEODOR'S SELF-UNDERSTANDING INTERVIEW

As our second tool for better understanding Teodor's perceptions of himself, we used the Self-Understanding Interview (Damon and Hart 1988).[72] This instrument situates children's responses to specific questions about their understanding of self as "me" (objective self) and as "I" (subjective self), in relation to the answers of other children their age. It measures understanding of self as "me" by categorizing children's statements into four self-schemes: physical, social, active, and psychological, and through determining the developmental level of each of these statements. It measures children's understanding of self as "I" in terms of agency, continuity, and distinctness of self from others.

According to this instrument, Teodor understands himself similarly to other children of his age. Most of his self-statements (nine out of nineteen) fell into the*psychological self-scheme* category,[73] which, according to Damon and Hart, means that Teodor defines himself mainly on the basis of his psychological characteristics or, in this case, his cognitive capacities. Most often, Teodor refers to himself as someone who knows about things—and who would like to know more. For example, he said, "I am a person who knows a lot about means of transportation," and also "I'll know math," or "I hope that I'll know everything, like, I'll know TTC and lots of things." He also said that he is smart—and that he would like to be even smarter. He said, "I am smart," and "I'd wanna be smart."

Teodor also made six self-statements that fell into the *social self-scheme* category.[74] Teodor's explanations of his self-statements most often referred to hisparents, followed by his friends, and bus drivers.[75] He made only one self-statement explicitly referring to his interpersonal relations ("Sometimes I behave bad and I lose friends"), but he made very detailed and consistent reference to himself as someone who might fulfill social roles and responsibilities on the job, especially as a knowledgeable and competent bus driver for the TTC.[76] Moreover, in explaining his answers that fell in other self-schemes, Teodor also often made reference to others, both real and imaginary (a critical factor in determining a developmental level of self-understanding, according to Damon and Hart).

There are three instances where Teodor refers to his *active self-scheme.*[77] For example, he said, "To be a bus-driver…I could get money when people pay their fare in the bus… But then I'd have to know how to drive a bus—like, what to push, like, when I am driving and I need to turn right, and I need to stop a little bit because of traffic."

Interestingly, only once did Teodor mention his *physical self-scheme.*[78] When asked whether he was different or the same five years ago, he said, "Maybe I was a little different because I was smaller and I knew less." He then continued to talk about what he meant by knowing less, and how his knowledge grew, but did not talk about his physical growth.[79]

With regard to Teodor's understanding of his own *agency*, he achieved level 3, meaning that he considers his agency to be due in part to communications and interactions with his parents. For example, when asked how he can become different, he says:

> Stop playing and start learning every day, without playing, until I know. And my parents ask me what I learned from yesterday—and the new questions—so like they ask me things one day, the next day they check if I know; if I don't know, next day they ask again. No. I learn again, and then they check again. And then they add new questions, then I repeat them again, so they see if I know and keep on doing that. And as soon as I become smart I could start playing.

Teodor also has a clear understanding of his being *distinct* from other people (there were two chunks that were scored in this category), in terms of his unique experiences and knowledge. For example, he says. "Nobody knows the same things that I know." Even more illustrative, when asked how he can be sure that he is different from everyone else when there are many people in the world he doesn't know, he replied, "Because, like, if I am in Bucharest and I ask someone, like, when I go to a subway station in Bucharest, and I ask, 'In Canada where does that bus go?' He wouldn't know that because for Canada he has to cross an ocean." We take this to show that he realizes that his unique subjective experiences have given him knowledge that others lack because they have not had them. This is clearly level 3, and possibly even level 4, according to Damon and Hart's scoring criteria.

Teodor showed a developmentally advanced understanding of his *continuity* over time. He has clear understanding of the relation between his earlier and his present characteristics, i.e., his evolving knowledge. He said, "I learn more. Like last year I didn't know *anything* [original emphasis] about Santa Clara buses and trains, but I learned some things about trains there." This interpretation is borne out even more clearly earlier in the interview, when Teodor is talking about how his understanding has changed and deepened as he has grown older, and how he has plans to learn new things in the future.

According to Damon and Hart (1988), each of the self-schemes can belong to one of four developmental levels of self-understanding.[80] When Teodor compared his knowledge of transportation systems to that of "real" bus drivers by saying "Some drivers don't know—for example, a TTC driver doesn't know schedules for Go Transit[81]—but I could easily know," he made a *comparative assessment* that belongs to the second developmental level and which emerges during mid-childhood (and is characterized by children's comparisons of themselves with other people). On the other hand, when he said, "I know lots, and I can easily help someone," he made a third level—*interpersonal implications*—statement that emerges in later childhood and early adolescence, and is recognizible by children's references to the manner of their interaction with others. Most of Teodor's responses fell into the second and third levels[82] and so his self-understanding is age-appropriate.

Reflections

Teodor's results on the Self-Understanding Interview show both similarities to and differences from those of other autistic children and adolescents matched on mental age[83] reported by Lee and Hobson (1998). Lee and Hobson found that their autistic participants' (aged 9–19; with verbal age range of 4; 4–9; 09) understanding of themselves significantly differed with regard to the *social aspect* of self (in both the number and quality of self-statements). Contrary to these children who made on average 1.5 such statements, Teodor made 6 self-statements in this category—which is more than the average number of such statements made even by non-autistic children in Lee and Hobson's study (5.6).[84] Lee and Hobson also reported that the number of self-statements at the third level (interpersonal implications) across all categories of self-statements was significantly lower in the autistic group than that in the comparison group (1.2 and 7.1, respectively). Teodor made 11 self-statements at this level and is clearly above the average range of nonautistic children in this respect. With regard to the quality of self-statements in the social category, Lee and Hobson reported that no autistic participants referred to a friend, whereas 70 per cent of control participants did so, and only 17 per cent of autistic participants mentioned families, as compared to 40 per cent of controls. Teodor, on the other hand, explicitly acknowledged his friends in his definition of self when he said that he is not proud of himself when he behaves badly and loses a friend. And although Teodor did not explicitly define himself in terms of his interactions with family members, he often referred to his family during the interview (i.e., 18 times).

It is certainly true that one reason for these differences could be the difference in the verbal abilities between Teodor and the autistic participants in Lee and Hobson's study. In fact, when we look at individual children's self-statements in this study, we find one participant that had five statements that belong to a social category—which is similar to Teodor—while most children had none. Unfortunately, we do not know other details about this participant, but it is reasonable to believe that the big differences in participants' age (both chronological and verbal) in the Lee and Hobson study contributed to the differences between our finding and theirs. The wide range of ages and abilities in this study may have also obscured developmental differences in self-understanding.

Teodor's self-statements also differed from those made by autistic participants in the Lee and Hobson study on three other aspects of self—active, physical, and psychological—both in number and quality. Autistic participants in the Lee and Hobson study referred most often to the *physical aspect* of self (mean 5.3); Teodor referred only once to this aspect of self. By contrast, Teodor most often referred to *psychological self* (i.e., nine times); Lee and Hobson's participants referred to this third most often (mean 2.8). And while all twelve autistic participants in the Lee and Hobson study together produced only two statements that referred to cognitive capacities ("I am a good thinker" and "I can do sums") (p.1138), Teodor alone made nine references to his cognitive capacities in his psychological scheme self-statements. In addition, none of the autistic participants in the Lee and Hobson study talked about preferences for psychological characteristics. In contrast, the overall tone of Teodor's interview and many of his explicit self-statements refer to his wish to be smarter than he perceives himself to be. And although, like autistic children in the Lee and Hobson study, Teodor did not refer to emotions when explicitly describing himself, he did mention them while explaining his self-statements. For example, in addition to an emotional incident with his mother, in which he cried, he also mentioned feelings of fun and boredom from his kindergarten years. Finally, while Teodor and autistic children in the Lee and Hobson study made a similar number self-statements that concern the active aspect of self (mean 3 and 3.3, respectively), Teodor referred to this aspect of self third most often, while autistic children in the Lee and Hobson study referred to it second most often.

In terms of Teodor's understanding of himself as subject, unlike the autistic children in Lee and Hobson's study, he is clearly at, and in some instances even above, his expected developmental level (level 3). Lee and Hobson found very few "chunks" (groups of statements that refer to the same self-characteristics) at level 3 (mean of 2.8); most striking, they found so few self-statements about the subjective selves of their subjects in response to specific questions that they considered their entire interviews, not just answers to the questions specifically designed by Damon and Hart to assess understanding of the subjective self. Of these responses, 94 per cent were scored at level 1 and 2; only two of the 12 autistic participants had a level 3 response. By contrast, Teodor's answers contained 10 relevant chunks, and these within the questions specifically designed to evaluate this dimension of self-understanding. In his answers, Teodor attained level 3 and even level 4.

Interestingly, Lee and Hobson noted that the autistic participants made reference to some unusually early autobiographical memories, which was not the case with the control group. Teodor too remembered some events that happened a while ago. For example, he remembered one emotional event with his mother (when he cried) when he was "a baby" (which, according to his mother, happened when he was less than four years of age). He also remembered one kindergarten event (when he was less than five years old), when he was "doing plop-plop-plop-plop...all day long" and annoyed all the other children.

One way to explain the differences found between how Teodor answered the Damon and Hart questions and how other autistic children assessed by Lee and Hobson answered may be that Teodor is diagnosed as having Asperger syndrome and therefore has better language skills. But perhaps autistic children do not answer these sorts of interview questions in the same way to anyone who asks them (in particular, when the initial question to the autistic child is "What kind of person is [child's name]?" as was the case in Lee and Hobson's study). The fact that Ljiljana has known Teodor for years, far from being a bias, may actually have allowed him to speak of things that he would not say to a near-total stranger. If true, this would be a methodological bias built into all studies of autism in which, in the name of scientific objectivity, the investigators do not get to know the autistic children personally.

Some other aspects of Teodor's self-statements were not relevant for the analysis according to Damon and Hart's protocol, but are especially important to look at in cases of atypical development. We conducted a content analysis of Teodor's self-statements which showed:

1. public transit was the most frequent theme in Teodor's interview
2. his self-statements often involved direct quotes, which gave the whole interview a dramatic tone
3. he never mentioned himself as being different from other children in any way (i.e., he did not make any reference to his autism).

RECURRING THEME

Thinking back to the accounts of Teodor by people who know him (his family and school staff, and even the psychiatrist), it is not at all unusual that most of his answers in this interview were related to public transit (i.e., 17 out of 20).[85] The only questions on which Teodor did not refer to his main interest were ones that asked about what he is *not*, or does not like about himself, or more specifically: What are you not like? What are you not proud of? and What do you like least about yourself? Thus, Teodor defines himself as a "person who *knows*[86] a lot about means of transportation and [is] *smart* on that." And he knows about "more than five transits in the world." He is also the most proud of his knowledge about different transits, so that he "can easily help someone." And of course "It would be good to be a bus driver" since he already knows where the buses go and the only thing to learn is how to drive a bus. When he was asked to compare himself as he is now with the baby he once was, he could only think of himself as somebody who "*didn't know anything* about buses." And as if he couldn't imagine himself without knowing anything about buses and trains, he added, "Maybe I knew a little bit." Finally, he believes that he knows about different transits more than bus drivers do, as "they don't know some things that I know." He pointed out, for example, that bus drivers in Toronto do not know about bus routes in nearby cities, but he does.

SPEECH CHARACTERISTICS

During this interview, when depicting social interactions with others, Teodor imitated the words and the tone of voice of his parents, two of his friends, children from the kindergarten, one teacher, Ljiljana, and some imaginary individuals such as bus drivers, passengers, children or just "somebody." For example, in one of his answers, Teodor made a reference to the conversation he had with his friend Victor, and made very dramatic changes in both the timbre and loudness of his voice:

> Sometimes [Victor] argues with me—I say, "This is ignored"—about his question—he says, "No, it's not ignored—what is it?" And I ignore him. "What

is it?" And I yell, "THIS IS IGNORED!"—loud—because he keeps and keeps and keeps and keeps on arguing.

AWARENESS OF THE "DIFFERENCE"

As far as his self-statements show, Teodor does not as yet see himself as being "different" from his peers, but we may take his statement that not many children want to play with him, as a beginning of this kind of awareness. This is important to know since some experts suggested that the life outcomes of autistic individuals might crucially depend on self-understanding and its motivating capacity for self-change (Bemporad 1979; Kanner 1973; Volkmar and Cohen 1985). We will return to this point later in the book.

These examples tell us something important about Teodor's self-understanding, and are important for our understanding of him as a person and his special way of being. Moreover, they give us some directions with regard to how to help him—and we will revisit these points later in this book.

We end this section by answering our initial question: Does Teodor understand himself? Teodor's self-perceptions as measured by the Damon and Hart interview are age-appropriate. Likewise, on Harter's Self-Perception Profile for Children, Teodor's assessment of his defining characteristics and his self-perceptions about these characteristics are echoed by accounts of others who know him well. It is true, however, that Teodor's self-evaluations of his "less important" competences on Harter's Self-Perception Profile for Children often differ from those of other people who evaluated him. For Simon Baron-Cohen and others, working from within the perspective of Theory of Mind deficit, these observed differences support their hypothesis that autistic persons do not understand their own minds. We disagree. Teodor's explanations were clearly supported by appropriate evidence and we believe that anyone considering things from his perspective would arrive at similar conclusions to Teodor about his competences.

Autistic brain: The neuro/biological perspectives

> Neurologic evaluation [of Teodor when he was approximately 6 years old] including a CT scan and EEG were normal... in February of 1997, he went on to have a right-sided seizure at school which lasted approximately 5 minutes, followed by several further seizures. He was hospitalized...and improved rapidly. Investigations at that time included an MRI scan of the head, as well as a SPECT scan. An EEG at the time showed some focal slowing in the left hemisphere that was thought to be postictal [i.e., post-seizure]. (Medical record of November 4, 1997)

The biological and neuroscientific perspectives are also important to understanding Teodor. These perspectives concern cell and brain features uniquely associated with autism. Specifically, they consider the etiology of autism (its causes), its neurological atypicalities (structural and functional), its neurophysiology, neuropsychology and neurochemistry.

Both Leo Kanner (1943, 1971) and Hans Asperger (1944/1991) suggested that autism is an organic condition. Nevertheless, when psychoanalysis was dominant, autism was considered a psychogenic disorder (i.e., caused by psychological factors), more specifically, by bad parenting (for a review of early views on autism see Rimland 1964). However, ever since the mid-sixties, autism has been recognized as a neuro/biological disorder. Bernard Rimland (1964) was the first to propose that a specific part of the brain—the reticular formation of the brain stem—is uniquely abnormal in autism, and responsible for its clinical manifestations. Currently, there is a general scientific agreement that autism has a neuro/biological basis; however, there is little agreement about what exactly this basis is. Here, we briefly review several lines of inquiry into what that biological basis might be.

The etiology of autism

Autism is currently conceptualized as a disorder with a heterogeneous etiology (i.e., it is caused by multiple factors acting together). Genetic and environmental factors, and their interactions, are thought to cause autism (for recent reviews see Folstein and Rosen-Sheidley 2001; Volkmar *et al.* 2004).

Strong evidence from twin and family studies suggests that autism has a genetic basis (Bailey *et al.* 1995).[87] It is currently commonly accepted that autism is caused by an interaction of several genes rather than by an action of a single gene (i.e., that it is a polygenic disorder; Folstein and Rosen-Sheidley 2001).[88] However, the actual genes involved in autism have not yet been identified (Veenstra-Vanderweele and Cook 2003; Volkmar *et al.* 2004). Several candidate genes involved in the development of the nervous system and the production of specific neurotransmitters have been investigated, but the replicability of findings has been low (Folstein and Rosen-Sheidley 2001; Philippe *et al.* 2002; Veenstra-Vanderweele and Cook 2003).[89] Several larger studies have also investigated candidate chromosomal regions that may contain one or more predisposing genes; these studies suggest that regions on chromosomes 2, 7, 15, 16 and X may be involved (Folstein and Rosen-Sheidley 2001; International Molecular Genetic Study of Autism Consortium 2001). However, all chromosomes but one—chromosome 14—have been reported as possibly contributing to autism (Gillberg 1998; Yonan *et al.* 2003).

All current genetic conceptualizations of autism include not only the characteristics of individuals with autism spectrum disorders, but also those of parents and siblings of autistic children who have autistic-like traits (such as preference for solitary activities, social and communication difficulties, and other traits of autism), but who do not meet the diagnostic criteria for any of the five disorders (i.e., who usually have only one or two of these traits). In other words, they emphasize its "broader phenotype" (Bolton *et al.* 1994; Le Couteur *et al.* 1996). However, it is still unknown whether all these conditions have a common genetic basis (Dawson *et al.* 2002; Folstein and Santangelo 2000; Volkmar *et al.* 2004). Susan Folstein and Susan Santangelo (2000) have recently reviewed the evidence that Asperger syndrome is genetically related to autism; however, only two recent studies specifically investigated the genetics of Asperger syndrome. One of these suggested involvement of chromosome 17 (Tentler *et al.* 2003), and the other identified regions on chromosomes 1, 3, 4, 6, 13 and 18 as possibly involved (Ylisaukko-oja *et al.* 2004).[90]

A number of environmental factors that might contribute to the development of autism have also been investigated. They include (1) obstetric complications (e.g., premature birth, low birth weight, respiratory distress syndrome, rhesus incompatibility, emergency cesarean section, resuscitation, severe fetal/neonatal infection, and severe trauma during birth); (2) intrauterine exposure to infections (e.g., to rubella, herpes encephalitis, cytomegalovirus, and influenza); (3) intrauterine exposure to drugs and chemicals such as alcohol, valproic acid,[91] and thalidomide,[92] and postbirth exposure to mercury[93] and vaccines; and (4) exposure to radiofrequency electromagnetic radiation (Bernard *et al.* 2001; Bolton *et al.* 1997; DeStefano *et al.* 2004; Kane 2004; Piven *et al.* 1993; Rodier 2000, 2004; Rodier and Hyman 1998). Although the findings about the role of these factors are mixed and difficult to interpret, most of them, as well as other general environmental factors, are believed to increase the risk of autism; however, it is not clear whether any of these factors is sufficient by itself to cause it (Bolton *et al.* 1997; Rodier and Hyman 1998).

Available evidence also suggests that many of the environmental factors can exert their influence only during a brief critical period. For example, thalidomide exposure has to occur between 20 and 24 days postconception (when the neural tube is closing) in order to produce autism (Rodier 2004). Currently research also suggests that some of the factors do not have the effect originally proposed; for example, a recent claim that the measles, mumps, and rubella (MMR) vaccination can cause autism in some children—based on anecdotal observations that received a lot of publicity (Wakefield *et al.* 1998)—was not supported by several recent controlled studies (DeStefano *et al.* 2004). In addition, most of the initial study's authors (10 of the 13 original authors) recently retracted their interpretation of the results of their study that suggested a possible link between MMR vaccine and autism (Murch *et al.* 2004). In their retraction they stated that they "wish to make it clear that in [the original] paper no causal link was established between MMR vaccine and autism as the data were insufficient" (p.750).

Finally, immune factors have also been suggested as playing a role in the development of autism. Several anomalies of immune system in autistic subjects have been reported, among them abnormal T cell activation, decreased relative numbers of helper-inducer lymphocytes, a lower helper-suppressor ratio, and antibodies against myelin basic protein (for a recent review see Krause *et al.* 2002). However, the results are conflicting and no clear picture of the role of immune factors in autism has emerged.

Neuroanatomical abnormalities

Studies that investigated brain abnormalities in autism have been deeply influenced by theories that postulate "core deficits." As there were many theoretical proposals of possible core deficits, a variety of brain abnormalities in support of them have been reported;[94] however, it should be noted that the replicability of specific findings has been relatively low and that there are many contradictory findings (for reviews, see Tanguay 2000; and Volkmar *et al.* 2004).[95] Neuroanatomical studies, which include structural magnetic resonance imaging (MRI)[96] and postmortem studies,[97] have shown that most major brain structures are in some way atypical.

In general, most studies found atypicalities in the following brain structures or areas:

1. limbic system—a collection of brain structures which include hippocampus, amygdala, parahippocampal and cingulate gyri; considered to be involved in processing of emotions and memory (Aylward *et al.* 1999); Bauman and Kemper 1994; Courchesne 1997)

2. cerebellum—thought to be involved in coordination of movement and modulation of cognitive processes[98] (Bauman and Kemper 1994; Courchesne *et al.* 1994; Piven, Saliba, Bailey and Arndt 1997)

3. brainstem—has many functions including modulation of sensory input (Bailey *et al.* 1998; Courchesne 1997; Hashimoto *et al.* 1992)

4. corpus callosum—a major tissue/band of nerve fibers connecting the left and right hemispheres (Egaas, Courchesne and Saitoh 1995;

Hardan, Minshew and Keshavan 2000; Piven, Bailey, Ranson and Arndt 1997)

5. cerebral cortex—the surface layer of the brain involved in higher cognitive functions such as final processing of sensations, voluntary movements, thought, reasoning, and memory (Bailey *et al.* 1998; Piven *et al.* 1990).

(For a recent review of structural MRI studies of brain anatomy in autism see Brambilla *et al.* 2003; for a review of postmortem studies see Bauman and Kemper 1994)

In addition, it has been found that the overall brain volume and weight tend to be increased in autistic persons, children in particular (a phenomenon called megalencephaly; Bailey *et al.* 1998; Bauman and Kemper 1994; Lainhart *et al.* 1997; Piven, Arndt, Bailey and Andreasen 1996). Recent studies have found that brain volume in autistic children appeared to be normal at birth, and that megalencephaly seems to develop during childhood (Courchesne *et al.* 2001; Courchesne, Carper and Akshoomoff 2003; Lainhart *et al.* 1997; Sparks *et al.* 2002). For example, Eric Courchesne and his colleagues (2001) found that brain volume of autistic children was average at birth but by 2 to 5 years of age had increased to be above average. Interestingly, this difference in brain volume was not found in older autistic children and adolescents. A similar finding, that brain volumes of autistic children 12 years old and younger, but not of children older than 12, were significantly different than those of typically developing children, was also reported by another research group (Aylward *et al.* 2002). A recent study also suggested that infantile macrocephaly (head circumference greater than 97th percentile—considered to be a consequence of megalencephaly) may be a risk factor for developing autism spectrum disorders (Bolton *et al.* 2001).

These findings provide some support for a new hypothesis about autism—the *brain growth dysregulation hypothesis*—that attempts to explain how the specific pattern of early abnormal neural development can lead to the specific anatomical and functional brain organization in later development (Akshoomoff, Pierce and Courchesne 2002; Courchesne *et al.* 2001). These findings show the importance of a neurodevelopmental perspective in studying autism and perhaps help explain some of the previously reported contradictory findings. They also show that not everybody is caught in the search for "the" core deficit in autism. As Greg Allen and Eric Courchesne (2001) recently suggested, echoing Hans Asperger's intuition, "There is clearly no 'core deficit' which at once characterizes and explains this complex condition. Rather, autism is a collection of multiple deficits resulting from multiple neural defects" (p.116). Fred Volkmar and his colleagues also make a similar point in a recent review (2004).

Linda Lotspeich and her colleagues (2004) also suggest that closer examination of patterns of multiple measures during development may shed light on neurodevelopmental differences between Autistic Disorder and Asperger's Disorder. However, so far there have been no replicable neuroanatomical differences that can distinguish between these two disorders. For example, Linda Lotspeich and her colleagues, in the first study that directly compared volumetric brain differences in cerebral gray matter of high-functioning autistic participants and those with Asperger syndrome, found no significant difference between them. Several studies that examined the amygdala volume of these two groups independently found that both subjects with Asperger syndrome (Haznedar *et al.* 2000) and high-functioning autistic subjects (Howard *et al.* 2000) had greater amygdala volume than normal. However, a previous study of amygdala volume in high-functioning autistic subjects found it to be lower than in the comparison group (Aylward *et al.* 1999).

Functional neuroimaging of autism

This line of research attempts to discover the association between brain structures and their functions by using techniques such as functional magnetic resonance imaging (fMRI), positron emission tomography (PET), and single photon emission computerized tomography (SPECT).[99] These studies reveal that—compared to control subjects—autistic subjects activate different (or differently activate) neural structures and/or pathways when they engage in cognitive tasks. So far, different brain activation has been reported in tasks of auditory perception and language (Boddaert *et al.* 2003; Muller *et al.* 1999), Theory of Mind tasks (Castelli *et al.* 2002; Frith 2001; Happé *et al.* 1996) and face perception (Critchley *et al.* 2000; Hubl *et al.* 2003; Pierce *et al.* 2001; Schultz *et al.* 2000).

For example, all recent studies of face processing in autistic subjects (all high-functioning autistic adults, or adults with Asperger syndrome) found that when looking at faces, autistic participants activated significantly less brain area typically involved in face perception (known as the fusiform gyrus).[100] However, the findings about the areas that were activated significantly more differ across studies, but usually include the brain area thought to be involved in perception of objects. When explaining these findings, researchers stress the use of alternate, and sometimes idiosyncratic, brain regions by autistic subjects (Pierce and Courchesne 2000) and the use of different strategies (Hubl *et al.* 2003).

Similarly, in several studies that measured brain activity while subjects performed different theory of mind tasks, autistic subjects and subjects with Asperger syndrome activated different brain regions than the control subjects (Happé *et al.* 1996), activated some regions less extensively than the control group (e.g., frontal lobes; Baron-Cohen *et al.* 1999) and failed to activate some structures such as amygdala (Baron-Cohen *et al.* 1999).

Functional imaging studies also revealed delayed maturation of the frontal cortex in autism (Zilbovicius *et al.* 1995), and temporal lobe dysfunction (Zilbovicius *et al.* 2000). However, for the most part functional neuroimaging studies of autism produced conflicting results and have not been able to consistently explain how the previously described structural brain abnormalities of autistic brains relate to functional brain abnormalities.

Neurophysiology of autism

This line of research has looked at electrical activity of the brain of autistic persons using electroencephalography (EEG). Findings of the EEG patterns of autistic persons' brains at rest have not been consistent, and no clear pattern of characteristics of autistic EEG waveforms has emerged. However, some interesting findings are obtained using an EEG technique called event-related potentials (ERP) that allows brain activity to be linked with different events such as stimulus presentation or motor movement, and with hypothesized psychological functions such as attention, cognition and working memory. The findings from these studies consistently show that brain wave components that are thought to reflect sensory and attentional processes and working memory context updating are usually delayed, absent or have smaller amplitudes in autistic subjects. For example, both auditory and visual processing have been found to be different in autistic than in control subjects—at both sensory and cognitive levels (e.g., Jansson-Verkasalo *et al.* 2003; Lincoln *et al.* 1993; Townsend, Harris and Courchesne 1996; Townsend *et al.* 2001; Verbaten *et al.* 1991). One of the most replicated findings is the smaller or absent P3b component of the ERP waves[101] generated by more posterior brain regions of the brain (i.e., parietal cortex). This component is hypothesized to reflect the updating of working-memory context (Donchin 1981; Polich and Kok 1995) and is attenuated or absent in autistic subjects in both auditory and visual modality (Courchesne *et al.* 1985; Novick *et al.* 1980).

Neuropsychology of autism

As mentioned in the previous section with regard to the executive function deficit hypothesis, neuropsychological tests such as the Wisconsin Card Sorting Test and the Tower of Hanoi have been useful in formulating and investigating this hypothesis. Efforts to differentiate high-functioning autism from Asperger syndrome on the bases of the neuropsychological tests of executive function have generated inconsistent findings, but generally seem to show no difference between the two conditions (Manjiviona and Prior 1999).

The pattern of performance of Asperger syndrome individuals on other neuro/psychological tests has also given rise to a new way of conceptualizing Asperger syndrome as the *right-hemisphere dysfunction* (Rourke 1995; Rourke *et al.* 1990; Rourke and Tsatsanis 2000). These studies have found that the pattern of performance of Asperger syndrome individuals on these tests resembles that of individuals with nonverbal learning disabilities (e.g., superior rote verbal memory and single word reading, and deficits in dealing with novel and complex material). The right-hemisphere dysfunction hypothesis has been supported by several neuropsychological and imaging studies (e.g., Gunter, Ghaziuddin and Ellis 2002; Klin *et al.* 1995; McKelvey *et al.* 1995). Finally, performance of autistic individuals on neuropsychological tests has provided the basis for yet another theory of autism as a disorder of *complex information processing* (Minshew *et al.* 1992; Minshew, Goldstein and Siegel 1997).

Neurochemistry of autism

Many studies have also investigated the levels of chemicals (such as neurotransmitters and neurotrophins) found in the brains of autistic subjects. Neurotrophins (also called growth factors) regulate neuronal growth, survival and connections during early brain development, and regulate the release of neurotransmitters, among other things, while neurotransmitters mediate communication within the nervous system throughout life.

One particular neurotransmitter, *serotonin*, has received the most attention. Serotonin plays a major role in the development of the central nervous system, social behavior, and emotion regulation, among other functions (Cook and Leventhal 1996; Jacobs and Azmitia 1992). Serotonergic receptors are particularly abundant in areas of the limbic system (Jacobs and Azmitia 1992), which are consistently found to be atypical in autistic subjects.[102] Concentrations of serotonin and its metabolites in autistic subjects have been measured in different body environments (i.e., blood, urine, and cerebrospinal fluid).[103] Most studies found elevated serotonin levels in the blood of autistic subjects (a phenomenon called hyperserotonemia; Anderson and Hoshino 1997; Cook and Leventhal 1996; Ritvo *et al.* 1970; Schain and Freedman 1961);[104] however, one study found that the level was decreased (Hérault *et al.* 1996), and one study that it was the same as in control subjects (Yuwiler *et al.* 1992). Levels of serotonin in urine of autistic subjects have been studied less extensively, and seem to be normal (Anderson and Hoshino 1997). Because of the invasive nature of measuring serotonin levels in the cerebrospinal fluid (involving lumbar puncture),[105] few studies have measured central serotonergic activity; but they found no difference between autistic and control subjects (Gillberg and Svennerholm 1987; Narayan *et al.* 1993).

A recent examination of the synthesis of brain serotonin in autism has added to these confusing findings, but possibly also brought some clarity, by noting the developmental aspect of serotonin synthesis, and the importance of studying serotonin in the brain rather than in the blood. Using positron emission tomography, Diane Chugani and her colleagues (1999) investigated developmental changes in serotonin synthesis in the brain of autistic children. Contrary to most studies just reviewed that found hyperserotonemia in autistic children's blood, this study found the opposite regarding the production of serotonin in the brain. In this study, the plateau values in the control group were 200 per cent of adult values while they were only 150 per cent of that value in the group of autistic children. Importantly, autistic children's capacity to synthesize serotonin seemed to have a different developmental course from that of children in the control group; while in the control group this capacity increased only until the age of five years and then declined toward adult values, in autistic children it increased gradually from two to fifteen years. From this data, Chugani and her colleagues concluded that developmental process in serotonin synthesis is disrupted in autistic children. Moreover, the same research group also found that different brain areas are differentially affected by altered serotonin synthesis, with the left hemisphere, basal ganglia and thalamus being more affected than the other areas (Chugani *et al.* 1997).[106] Although significant, these results have yet to be replicated; moreover, since the control participants were children with epilepsy, the interpretation of these results also must be approached with caution.

The neurotransmitter *dopamine*—which has a role of modulating attention, perception, motor activity, and social behavior—has also been implicated in autism. However, the evidence of its dysfunction in autism is inconclusive, with some studies finding elevated levels of dopamine precursors in the brains of autistic subjects (e.g., Gillberg and Svennerholm 1987), and other studies finding no differences (e.g., Narayan *et al.* 1993; for a review see Anderson and Hoshino 1997). The evidence for a possible involvement of the neurotransmitter *norepinephrine*—with a role in arousal, attention, filtering of irrelevant stimuli, anxiety, and learning—is also inconclusive (Anderson and Hoshino 1997). There is also some evidence that autistic subjects have an atypical *GABAergic system*—which has an important role in the early development of the central nervous system (Blatt *et al.* 2001; Fatemi *et al.* 2002). A few studies found that when compared with the blood plasma of the control subjects, blood plasma of autistic subjects has lower concentrations of a neuropeptide[107] *oxytocin*—which has an important role in the regulation of social behavior (Green *et al.* 2001; Modahl *et al.* 1998).

Levels of *neurotrophins*[108] have also been investigated in autistic subjects. There is some initial evidence of elevated blood levels of four neuropeptides and neurotrophins (Nelson *et al.* 2001). However, these findings have yet to be replicated and their importance established since autistic children were not distinguishable from those with mental retardation with regard to any of the studied substances.

Studies of neurochemistry in autism may have important implications for treatment of autism; however, so far there have been no autism-specific pharmacological treatments, although serotonin- and dopamine-related drugs have been reported to be effective at reducing behavioral symptoms of autism such as repetitive and compulsive behaviors in some autistic individuals in some, but not all, studies (McDougle and Posey 2002; Volkmar *et al.* 2004). However, most of these studies have serious methodological limitations such as lack of control for placebo effect, questionable outcome measures, and small numbers of subjects (Tsai 1999). Most importantly, safety of these drugs has not yet been established, and many adverse effects have been reported in children before puberty in particular (McDougle and Posey 2002; Tsai 1999). Therefore, at present, it seems that the numerous side effects reported in all studies outweigh some reported improvements. In our opinion, such drugs should not be used before their effectiveness and safety have been fully established.

In sum, neuroscientific studies of autism have identified a variety of abnormalities in brain areas associated with specific psychological functions found to be impaired in psychological studies of autism (e.g., emotion, executive function, theory of mind, language, and memory). However, since the replicability of findings has been low, it has been repeatedly noted that we need a more precise characterization of autism, and better control for age and intelligence differences (Koenig, Tsatsanis and Volkmar 2001; Lotspeich *et al.* 2004; Volkmar *et al.* 2004). For all these reasons, the neuroscientific search for causes and neural bases of autism has so far not been very successful. We still do not know the structural, functional and/or biochemical events that cause autism, how it develops, and when, how—or even whether—it should be treated.

TEODOR'S BRAIN: NO SPECIFIC ABNORMALITIES

Teodor has been evaluated neuroscientifically using different tests, ever since he was seven-and-a-half years old. He was first tested when he was admitted to the emergency room "with a picture suggestive of acute confusional migraine or seizures."[109] The neurological exam he received at that time (which included an examination of cranial nerves, reflexes, motor tone and strength, sensation and gait) was normal (except for a knee jerk that was absent on the left side and 1+ in other extremities). His CT scan at that time was normal and his EEG was "within normal limits" (EEG Report, September 9, 1996). Finally, a chromosomal analysis, including a test for fragile-X, was conducted on Teodor's blood: the results were negative.

About five months later, Teodor had a seizure episode for which he had to be hospitalized (as described in the psychiatric perspective). It was at that time that Teodor was diagnosed as having Asperger's Disorder. During his hospital stay, he was also evaluated using several neurological tests. In addition to the neurological exam, an EEG and MRI and SPECT scans were performed. Teodor's MRI scan was described as "very detailed, specifically looking for a hypothalamic hamartoma[110] as well as for other focal cortical abnormality" and was found to be "completely normal" (February 14, 1997). However, his SPECT scan showed "decreased perfusion [i.e., blood flow] of the temporal lobes somewhat worse on the left. As well, there [was] asymmetric activity at the basal ganglia, possibly slightly increased on the left and probably slightly decreased on the right" (February 12, 1997). The neurologist, however, noted that the SPECT scan abnormality was "very subtle and not fully convincing. If a real finding, the significance is unclear, as such a deficit has not been described about Asperger's to our knowledge." Teodor's EEG record showed asymmetrical background and "some focal slowing [in] the left hemisphere." The neurologist's conclusion was that there was nothing specifically abnormal about Teodor's brain other than some postseizure activity (i.e., "some focal slowing [in] the left hemisphere" seen in an EEG record). It was recommended that these tests be repeated.

In three-and six-month follow-ups (April and June 1997), Teodor was tested again using the same procedures and the findings were almost unchanged: his EEG record showed some left hemisphere "disturbances;" his SPECT scan revealed a decreased blood flow to both temporal lobes and alterations to basal ganglia; and the MRI scan was normal. The neurologist's interpretation of these results was that Teodor "does not have an obvious etiology. Although the EEG and SPECT scans are abnormal, these lesions are not apparent on recent MRIs. Thus, it appears that [Teodor] has functional as opposed to structural abnormality."

Several more follow-up examinations were performed, but no new information was obtained other than an apparent normalization of his EEG, leading to Teodor's discontinuation of seizure medication. Teodor's EEGs improved over time and were only "mildly abnormal" with the "left temporal sharp waves [being] potentially epileptiform" (i.e., resembling epilepsy) on March 11, 1998. By February 24, 2000, his EEG was "within normal limits".

Commentary and reflections

Even a superficial look at findings about Teodor's brain highlights both the complexity of autistic neuroanatomy and neurophysiology and immaturity of our current neuroscientific methods. According to two of these methodologies, the CT and MRI scans, Teodor's brain is just fine, while according to two other, SPECT scan and EEG, it is not quite so—although supposedly only because of his seizures and not his autism. Discrepancies between results of different methodologies, SPECT and MRI scans in particular, have already been reported in autistic literature. For example, a study that directly compared SPECT and MRI scans of 23 autistic children found that while MRI scans of all the children were normal, 20 children had abnormal SPECT scans (Ryu *et al.* 1999). Ryu and colleagues suggested that the SPECT scans may be more sensitive for revealing physiological abnormalities in autism than the MRI.

However, studies that used only SPECT scans to investigate autistic brains produced highly inconsistent results ranging from no cortical abnormalities (Zilbovicius *et al.* 1992), to abnormalities in different brain areas (such as temporal, frontal, parietal and occipital lobes; cerebellum, thalami, and basal ganglia; Chiron *et al.* 1995; George *et al.* 1992; Gillberg *et al.* 1993; Mountz *et al.* 1995; Ohnishi *et al.* 2000; Ryu *et al.* 1999; Starkstein *et al.* 2000). Importantly, most of these studies found reduced activity in the temporal lobes (usually together with some other abnormalities)—just as in Teodor's SPECT scan. However, some studies found this reduced activity in both temporal lobes (e.g., Gillberg *et al.* 1993; Ohnishi *et al.* 2000), some in the left (e.g., Chiron *et al.* 1995; Starkstein *et al.* 2000), and some in the right (e.g., George *et al.* 1992). In his first SPECT scan, Teodor had reduced blood flow in both temporal lobes, although this was more pronounced in the left. This pattern most resembles the results of James Mountz and his colleagues' study (1995) in which reduced activity was found in both temporal lobes, but somewhat more reduced in the left. Importantly, this group of researchers also found decreased activity in the right basal ganglia, which is another site of altered activity identified in Teodor's scan. However, Mountz and colleagues also found reduced activity in the parietal lobes, which was not the case with Teodor's SPECT scan.[111] Interestingly, Teodor's subsequent SPECT scans showed reduced activity only in the temporal lobes (both left and right), which is the pattern found in two other SPECT studies (Gillberg *et al.* 1993; Ohnishi *et al.* 2000).

What is the relevance of all these findings? What do they tell us about Teodor? Unfortunately, the answer seems to be "not much," at least for now. This is because, given the current state of scientific knowledge, it is hard to interpret them. We know that the temporal lobes are crucial for normal speech and language development, for processing of sensory information, and for regulating emotion, memory, learning, and social interaction (Gloor 1997). However, decreased blood flow in the temporal lobes is not specific to autism. It is also found in temporal lobe epilepsy (Rowe *et al.* 1991) and language disorders (Yang *et al.* 2002). A decreased blood flow in the basal ganglia (a collection of nuclei with a crucial role in creating and controlling movement) is also associated with seizures (Sojkova *et al.* 2003) and obsessive-compulsive disorder (Lucey *et al.* 1997).

We know that Teodor has difficulties with social interactions and language and that he has specific affinity for "funny" sounds. He also "has an obsession" with the public transit system. It is tempting to speculate that the pattern of dysfunction in the two areas of Teodor's brain, temporal lobes (associated with social interactions, language, and sound processing) and the basal ganglia (associated with obsessions) may be responsible for his autism. However, this would be too simplistic an interpretation, in particular because most SPECT studies of autistic subjects did not find alterations in the basal ganglia.[112] Therefore, it seems more likely that this pattern of dysfunction is more related to Teodor's seizures than to his autism. This interpretation is supported by the results of his follow-up SPECT scans (when his seizures started to improve) in which there was no mention of basal ganglia. Moreover, autistic subjects in Mountz and colleagues' study also appear to have had seizures.[113] The significance of hypoactivation of Teodor's temporal lobes, even after his seizures improved, still needs to be explained and may well be related to his autism. However, in spite of a number of independent reports of both structural (e.g., Bailey *et al.* 1998; Bauman and Kemper 1994) and functional (other than in SPECT studies, e.g., Zilbovicius *et al.* 2000) atypicalities of autistic temporal lobes, the specific mechanism by which they may be involved in autism is still not known. Moreover, in most studies, temporal lobes are not the sole area of atypicalities, as was also true of Teodor's SPECT scans. Finally, even if Teodor's atypical temporal lobes are responsible for his social and language difficulties and his atypical processing of auditory stimulation, it is not at all clear what the practical implication of this would be—how we could intervene differently to help him, given this knowledge.

In spite of numerous biological and neuroscientific studies of autism (around 7000 articles worldwide; Volkmar *et al.* 2004), and many structural and functional atypicalities that were found in autistic brains, it is still unclear how they may explain the behavior and experience of autistic persons. One part of the difficulty lies in the fact that we still do not know enough about how a typical brain works. Another part of the problem is the inconsistent definitions of autism across studies. Third is the methodological problems of most studies that include small sample size, lack of adequate control group, and lack of control for numerous contributing (and confounding) factors, such as other neurological and psychological conditions such as seizures and mental retardation. For example, we still do not know whether underlying mechanisms differ in autistic individuals with and without mental retardation, and until we do know this, we should not mix them in the same group. Given all these limitations it is not at all surprising that results of neuroscientific investigations of autism (as well as previously described psychiatric and psychological ones) are inconclusive. However, the contradictory findings of neuroscientific investigations of autistic subjects show once more the importance of careful consideration of developmental, behavioral, and cognitive—including experiential—characteristics of autistic subjects taking part in these investigations. We believe that once we start paying attention to the multiple levels of differences among autistic subjects, we will start getting a much clearer picture of how, perhaps various, brain abnormalities in the developing autistic brain act to produce autistic behavior and cognition including experience. It is only when the multiple levels of differences among subjects are taken into account that the conflicting results we now have will start making sense.

The neuroscientific perspective might have important implications for early identification of autism and for the design of pharmacological treatments to "cure" it. However, higher-functioning autistic persons strongly express the view that if they could choose whether or not to be autistic, they would want to be autistic (see Grandin 1995a; Holliday Willey 1999; Sinclair 1993). This leads us to consider a final, very different, subjective perspective on autism.

5

A Transfer Boy

The First-Person Perspective[114]

For the last 20 years many persons diagnosed as "having" high-functioning autism or Asperger syndrome have written books and articles and spoken publicly about their life experiences, and about what it means to be autistic (Barron and Barron 2002; Carpenter 1992; Grandin 1984, 1992, 1995a, 1995b, 1997, 2000; Grandin and Scariano 1986; Holliday Willey 1999; Jackson 2002; Jolliffe, Lansdown and Robinson 1992; Miedzianik 1986; Schneider 1999; Sinclair 1992, 1993; Williams 1992, 1994, 1996b, 1998). Without any intention to make a comprehensive review of these writings (a project in itself), we will briefly review some of the common themes most relevant for the issues discussed in this book that are found in some of the most well-known examples of autobiographical writings of autistic persons.

What is autism?

First and foremost, autistic persons—without exception—feel misunderstood by scientists. For example, Liane Holliday Willey, a doctor of education, writer and researcher, writes, "Autism touches many, and yet, it is one of the most misunderstood developmental disorders" (1999, p.13). Edgar Schneider, a retired mathematician and computer programmer, writes in his autobiography, "I hope that I have been able to give some ideas of what autism is all about, because it has to be the most misunderstood disability there is" (1999, p.116). For Jim Sinclair, a rehabilitation counselor, disability educator and consultant, one of the founders and the coordinator of the first "autistic-run self-help and advocacy organization for autistic people"—Autism Network International (ANI),[115] being autistic means that:

> What is normal for other people is not normal for me, and what is normal for me is not normal for other people. In some ways I am terribly ill-equipped to survive in this world, like an extraterrestrial stranded without an orientation manual. (1992, p.302)

He adds, "But my personhood is intact. My selfhood is undamaged. I find great value and meaning in my life, and have no wish to be cured of being myself" (Sinclair 1992, p.302). He also protests: "Autism is not an appendage:"

> Autism isn't something a person has, or a "shell" that a person is trapped inside. There's no normal child hidden behind the autism. *Autism is a way of being.* It is pervasive; it colours every experience, every sensation, perception, thought, emotion, and encounter, every aspect of existence. *It is not possible to separate the autism from the person*—and if it were possible, the person you'd have left would not be the same person you started with. (1993, 'Autism is not an appendage', para. 1, emphases added)

Donna Williams, an artist, teacher, and counselor, author of six books (three of which are autobiographies), also diagnosed as autistic, expresses her views in the following way:

> Autism is a label which describes outer behaviours, not inner realities. It can appear, disappear and reappear in varying degrees in different circumstances. In other words, depending on strategies and adaptations, it can exist even though it is not apparent and, as appearances can also be misleading, it can appear where it is not in fact experienced. The word autism is, therefore, less substantial, less dependable, than a piece of lint, and I've always tried to express this by using the word enclosed within inverted commas; 'autism', rather than Autism. 'Autism' as an experience describes a very complex interplay between identity, personality, environment, experience and the equipment with which to integrate and make sense of that experience. 'Autism' is simply an internal human 'normality' with the volume turned up. We all have experienced moments when we aren't quite aware or when we are too aware to handle the world. Or moments when we aren't quite aware of the company we are in or so overly aware of it that it gets hard to function. We all have had times when we've had hardly any awareness of our bodies, even been out of them, or felt so in, weighed down by them, that we become hypercritical, eager to escape, tune out, disappear. We have all had times when we've lost the plot, the why, the what or been distracted by the meta-reality inside our heads to the extent that we are suddenly jolted out of a daydream. So too, have we all had moments when we have been so aware that we have taken things in almost overwhelming, extreme detail. For me, the experience of 'autism' is not of any of these things in themselves, but rather the frequency and extremity with which they are experienced and the *degree* to which these experiences affect

> how one expresses oneself and relates to one's inner world and the outer world. It's a matter of whether you visit these states or whether you've lived there. (1998, pp.9–10)

Donna Williams addresses other scientific misconceptions about autism. She believes that:

> Those seeking to test people with 'autism' might begin by daring to imagine that these people may not be *lesser-developed versions of non-autistic people* but, rather, people who HAVE developed, sometimes substantially, along a very different track from non-autistic people. Looking at how 'autistic' people measure up to non-autistic people according to a non-autistic developmental path tells the researcher nothing about how far the same person may have developed a whole range of adaptations, compensations and strategies along an 'autistic' track. (1996a, p.235, emphasis added)

Even thirteen-year-olds with Asperger syndrome feel that professionals should listen more to what they have to say about themselves and their autism. One of these young people, Luke Jackson, author of the book, *Freaks, Geeks and Asperger Syndrome: A User Guide to Adolescence,*[116] writes:

> Another big reason for writing this [book] was the hope that professionals of any sort may read it and begin to understand the many, many people who are similar to me. / So, if you are a professional, don't just put this down and think that I am just a sweet kid. Please read on and learn more. (2002, p.14)

He adds:

> A lot of people seem to think that AS [Asperger syndrome] people do and say the most nonsensical things. I must say that people who don't have AS do many things that don't make sense to me! (p.106)

Sensory sensitivities[117]

All autistic persons who wrote their autobiographies wrote about their heightened sensory experiences. They wrote about their (hyper- and hypo-) sensitivities in almost all sensory modalities (e.g., visual, auditory, tactile, kinesthetic and olfactory). However, different individuals describe different patterns (i.e., strongly liking or disliking some kinds of stimuli in different modalities). In general, most of them do not like, and tend to avoid whenever possible, certain visual, auditory and tactile stimuli such as loud noises, being touched, or touching certain objects (Grandin 1992, 1995a; Grandin and Scariano 1986; Holliday Willey 1999; Williams 1992, 1994, 1996b, 1998). Liane Holliday

Willey wrote, "As much as I loved to chew scratchy and gritty textures, I often found it impossible even to touch some objects. I hated stiff things, satiny things, scratchy things, things that fit me too tightly" (1999, p.25).

Interestingly, many of these individuals find voices and/or words to be particularly fascinating. For example, Donna Williams (1999a) writes, "I chattered incessantly to myself, annoying everyone else. People said that I simply loved the sound of my voice" (p.28). Anne Carpenter, another autistic person, says, "I like the sound of my own voice" (Dewey 1991, p.204).[118] Temple Grandin also wrote, "I talked and talked and talked" (Grandin and Scariano 1986, p.85). Autistic persons have also written about the visual and kinesthetic features of words or production of voices. For example, Donna Williams (1996a) wrote about "words that had good visual patterns, words that had felt good in my mouth, words that had sounded good to my ears" (p.243). Liane Holliday Willey (1999) too wrote about auditory and kinesthetic features of spoken words. She said, "I loved the way most words played on my tongue. I loved the way they caused different parts of my mouth to move" (p.24).

Other autistic persons have also reported that sounds elicited experiences in one or more other senses (e.g., vision, taste, smell)—a phenomenon called synesthesia:

> Sounds are often accompanied by vague sensations of colour, shape texture, movement, scent or flavour. It is as if information was received in several modes even though the signal comes from one source. (Cesaroni and Garber 1991)

Making order out of chaos

Almost all autistic persons who have written about themselves have also written about the confusion and unpredictability of the world, and their search for order. When Jerry Goldsmith (a pseudonym) was a child, he experienced the world mainly as confusion and terror: "Everything was unpredictable and strange"—except labels and prices in grocery stores (Bemporad 1979, p.192). Therese Jolliffe, an autistic person who has a doctoral degree in psychology, writes, "A large part of my life is spent just trying to work out the pattern behind everything. Set routines, times and rituals all help to get order into an unbearably chaotic life" (Jolliffe *et al.* 1992, p.16). Most autistic persons found the first signs of predictability in letters, numbers and patterns of sounds. Donna Williams writes:

> I LOVED TO copy, create, and order things. I loved our set of encyclopedias. They had letters and numbers on the side, and I was always checking

> to make sure they were in order or putting them that way. I was making order out of chaos. (1999a, p.42)

She also writes, "I loved letters and learned them quickly. Fascinated by the way they fitted together into words, I learned those, too" (p.28). However, she also describes her difficulty in understanding the meaning of what was said to her, since people's words were for her just "a pattern of sounds" (p.9). Similarly, Liane Holliday Willey wrote:

> I did find solace in the dark print so neatly typed on the white pages. I enjoyed the rhythmic pattern and the flow that moved the eye from left to right, from top to bottom. I welcomed the routine that insisted I stop for periods and break for commas and new paragraphs. (1999, p.24)

Sean Barron sums it up: "I hated change, all change! I loved repetition" (Barron and Barron 2002, p.206).

All-absorbing interests

Autistic persons write about their strong need to do certain things (usually related to the predictable aspects of the world such as words, numbers, labels, or any other patterns) to the exclusion of most (and occasionally all) other aspects of the world. In many cases these interests lead to successful careers. For example, Sean Barron recollects his early interests:

> I had an intense interest in dead-end streets. The things I liked to do, in general, were those that offered some variation but were still repetitious. So dead-end streets were perfect. I knew the different ways that such street[s] could look—two neighboring streets could both be dead-ends but look and feel totally unlike each other. Yet they both ended, and in that way they were the same. (Barron and Barron 2002, p.89)

Sean Barron also had an interest in school buses:

> I love the sameness of all the buses—they were all the same colour and had the same words on them—but there were minute differences too; for instance, the number on each was different, and there were differences also in the shapes of the "noses" (some very pointed, others rather blunted). My goal was to see all the buses the school owned in one year so I could compare all of them. I loved the way they looked when they were all parked in a line, and I got very angry when bus 24 was late and I had to go home before I saw it. It was not supposed to do that! It was supposed to be in that line with the other buses. (Barron and Barron 2002, p.108)

Autistic persons also write about their need to talk about their interests. For example, Temple Grandin wrote, "If a particular topic intrigued me, I zeroed in on that subject and talked it into grounds. It was no wonder I was nicknamed 'Chatterbox'" (Grandin and Scariano 1986, p.31).

When describing his "specialist interest", computers, Luke Jackson writes, "I feel an overwhelming excitement in me that I cannot describe. I just have to talk about it and irritation at being stopped can easily develop into raging fury" (2002, p.44). Older autistic persons write about alternative ways to meet this need, as the following conversation between two of them, Anne Carpenter and Jack Dewey, recorded by Jack's mother, illustrates:

Anne: I sometimes drive my mother up the wall by talking too much about the same subject.

Jack: Oh, yes, I have quite a number of things I talk about and can't let go of. But since you've [refers to his mother] conditioned me not to bore people, I talk to myself incessantly.

Anne: Oh, I talk to myself all the time, too! (Dewey 1991, p.204)

One of Jack's interests is music (he is a piano tuner), an interest shared with other autistic persons (e.g., David Miedzianik, Edgar Schneider and Donna Williams). Other common interests include writing—including poetry (Liane Holliday Willey, David Miedzianik, Jim Sinclair, Donna Williams), psychology, counseling and rehabilitation (Sean Barron, Temple Grandin, Liane Holliday Willey, Therese Jolliffe, Jim Sinclair, Donna Williams), computers (Luke Jackson and Edgar Schneider), mathematics (Edgar Schneider), animal science and design of animal facilities (Temple Grandin), and linguistics and politics (Liane Holliday Willey). All these and other common interests (e.g., history, library science) have also been reported in clinical accounts and life outcome studies of autistic adults (Attwood 1998; Howlin *et al.* 2004; Hurlbutt and Chalmers 2002; Mercier, Mottron and Belleville 2000; Wing 1981).

A need to be alone vs. a need to be with others

Autobiographical writings show that not all autistic persons have the same social needs. Some of them write about a desire to be with others, while others write about the need for privacy. For example, David Miedzianik, at the age of 28, said, "I wish I could meet someone that I could get married to" although, "I don't know if I like the idea of living with someone" (1986, p.58). Later he added, "Well recently I have got so fed up with no-one going out with me that I keep putting adverts in magazines" (p.65). When ads in the magazines did not work, he did not get discouraged:

> Recently in about this last year or so I have been writing letters to the radio; I have had my letters read out on Radio One quite a bit. I keep thinking if I get things read out on the radio I might make some new friends. Things really get me down, wandering around Rotherham most of the time by myself. Not having any girls that like me really makes me sad. (p.95)

Donna Williams writes about the need to be with others—but under particular conditions: "The only thing I was missing was inclusion, and when I wanted this I wanted it on my terms, so I could throw it away at some later date, as though friendship was an apple gone bad" (1992, p.34).

On the other hand, in spite of having friends, others write about their primary need for privacy. For example, Jack Dewey said, "I don't suffer from loneliness...I seem to crave a lot of privacy" (Dewey 1991, p.203). Similarly, Holliday Willey wrote:

> When I think of my earliest years, I recall an overwhelming desire to be away from my peers. I much preferred the company of my imaginary friends. Penny and her brother Johnna were my best friends, though no one saw them but me. (1999, p.18)

And later, she adds:

> I rarely remember a time, best friends in the background or not, when I did not prefer to be alone. Unlike most people I knew, I did not grow up feeling the need to make deep and strong connections with others. I do not think I ever consciously sought a friend or disregarded a friend. I was nice to people I knew and friendly to people I only passed in the halls. (p.41)

Jim Sinclair, who believes himself to be "capable of making authentic connections" and to have "exactly as many relationships as [he] want[s]," (1992, p.301) writes:

> I can be very interested in individuals once I've met them, but I don't feel a need to have relationships in the absence of specific people to relate to. During school breaks I can go for days or weeks without any personal contact with other human beings, and I may get bored, but I don't get lonely. I don't need social contact. (1992, p.300)

Likewise, Edgar Schneider writes:

> I have never felt lonely or a need for what could be called "the warmth of another human being," even a loving woman, or a good friend of either sex. I have very much enjoyed the company of those with whom I could

> have an interesting and stimulating conversation, but not, as so many other people seem to be able to do, simply because he or she is "a good person"... Yet, with people who fervently share interests with me, I have been able to form very close friendships. (1999, p.57)

In a similar vein, Temple Grandin writes, "I had a few friends who were interested in the same things, such as skiing and riding horses. Friendship always revolved around what I did rather than who I was" (1995b, p.132). Referring to the lack of close relationship in her life, she said:

> I know that things are missing in my life, but I have an exciting career that occupies my every waking hour. Keeping myself busy keeps my mind off what I may be missing. Sometimes parents and professionals worry too much about the social life of an autistic adult. I make social contacts via my work. If a person develops her talents, she will have contacts with people who share her interests. (1995b, p.139)

On the diagnosis of autism

Everyone whose writings we reviewed believes strongly that parents of children diagnosed as autistic should tell their children that they are autistic and what it means (Sinclair 1992). This belief comes from their own experience of great relief they felt when they learned that there are other children/people like them.[119] They also believe that this knowledge can be a driving force of self-change.

After seeing the movie about an autistic boy, *Son Rise*, sometime during his high-school years, Sean Barron, who has a degree in Early Childhood, asked his mother, "Mom, I'm autistic too, aren't I?" He, for the first time saw the possibility that perhaps "what made me like this was a disease of some kind and that I was not a horrible person after all" (Barron and Barron 2002, p.229)—which was something that he had feared for some time. Donna Williams learned about autism at age 25 and it "helped explain [her] world" (1999b, p.8). Eugene Thomas (pseudonym) "never knew what was wrong" with him and thought he was "the only one in the world like this" (Hurlbutt and Chalmers 2002, p.105).

Anne Carpenter (a librarian mentioned in the previous section) discovered her autism after reading Temple Grandin's book:

> I read the book, and all the fixations, the repetitive conversations about the same topic, and the weird mannerisms came back to me. It was as if my whole personality were contained in the pages of that book! Upset, but also relieved, I knew that this was it—I was definitely autistic... I was officially diagnosed as having autism... *That diagnosis was to be the force that would change my life.* Now that there was a name for that monstrous problem I had been carrying around for years, maybe I could find ways to eliminate at

> least some of the odd and socially unappealing behaviors. (1992, p.293, emphasis added)

Thirteen-year-old Luke Jackson could not agree more. He writes that not knowing his diagnosis "was a million time[s] worse than you can ever imagine" (2002, p.25). Here is his description of his discovery that followed reading an article in *The Guardian* that his mother just happened to place in front of him "as if she had done it by accident" (p.34):

> I was twelve years old when I read this article... As I read through the article my first reaction was relief. It was [as] if I had a weight lifted off my shoulders... I read it and reread it, and said to Mum, "Do you think I could have AS [Asperger syndrome]?" (p.34)

And he continues:

> I had finally found the reason why other people classed me as weird. It was not just because I was clumsy or stupid. My heart lightened instantly and the constant nagging that accompanied me all my life (not my Mum) stopped immediately. I finally knew why I felt different, why I felt as if I was a freak, why I didn't seem to fit in. Even better, it was not my fault! At first I wanted to run out and tell the world. I felt like charging out into the streets and shouting, "Hey, look at me, I have Asperger syndrome. I am not a freak." (p.34)[120]

Therefore, Luke urges, "I personally think that a child *should* be told and the sooner the better. Believe me I know!" (2002, p.30, emphasis original). He adds:

> I can't stress enough how bugged I was to "discover" my AS. At least five years after I was actually diagnosed. Mum could have saved me a lot of years of worry because I always knew I was different. (p.35)

Finally, Luke raises an important ethical point—that of children's rights:

> If a child gets taken to see doctors and other people and the parents talk in whispered conversations about them and tell the child nothing, then that is denying the child the *right to know* about themselves. (p.37, emphasis added)

View about intervention strategies

Autistic persons express their concern about some interventions designed to help them. For example, Donna Williams writes:

> It is important to recognize the risks of chronic stress in training people to function in the absence of being able to feel for, identify with, or experi-

> ence their own functioning. This can be like starvation of the soul. It is important that people still know who they are inside, whether high or low functioning and it is important that people get to be who they are for at least some designated part of every day even if it means they sit there doing nothing, rock or play with buttons. (1996a, p.104)

In general, autistic persons are proud of being autistic (Grandin, Holliday Willey, Sinclair, Williams) and do not wish for a cure for autism. For example, Liane Holliday Willey writes:

> Yet, no matter the hardships, I do not wish for a cure to Asperger's Syndrome. What I wish for, is a cure for the common ill that pervades too many lives; the ill that makes people compare themselves to a normal that is measured in terms of perfect and absolute standards, most of which are impossible for anyone to reach. I think it would be far more productive and so much more satisfying to live according to a new set of ideals that are anchored in far more subjective criteria, the fluid and affective domains of life, the stuff of wonder...curiosity...creativity...invention...originality. Perhaps then, we will all find peace and joy in one another. (1999, pp.121–122)

Role of self-control: Self-intervention

However, the above statements should not be taken as autistic persons' acceptance of autism as a total controller of their lives either. Instead, autistic persons want to be in control of their thoughts and actions—their lives. Sean Barron writes:

> I took a look at myself in a way I had never done before, and this is what I saw; I had problems, real ones, big ones. But that didn't mean that there was something fundamentally wrong with me, that I was unlike everybody else in the world. I knew that I was separate from my problems I had and that I could overcome them. I declared war! I was going to fight against all the behaviors I had obeyed all my life... Dead-end streets and bus numbers still went round and round in my head, and I pushed them out—I made myself think other thoughts instead. (Barron and Barron 2002, p.232)

But this is of course not an easy thing to do. Donna Williams writes about her almost lifelong battle with her autistic habits (i.e., compulsions) that started when she was twelve). When she was in her thirties, she was still fighting, with no signs of giving up:

> I CAN FIGHT AUTISM...I WILL CONTROL IT...IT WILL NOT CONTROL ME. (1996b, p.207)

In her book *Somebody Somewhere*, she describes her life as a "journey from 'my world' to 'the world,' in which I took the reins out of the hands of my autism and took control of my life" (1996b, p.5). She describes this process as hard and long work involving not only determination to succeed but also "asking the right people the right questions, once you knew what they were" (1996b, p.3).

Thirteen-year-old Luke Jackson has just started the journey of self-intervention:

> I try to find a balance between making an effort to mix with others without standing out too much, and accepting the inevitable—that I am always going to seem a little different. I am not sure whether I do a good job of this. (2002, p.30)

Commentary

From the perspective of those who are living autism—and are able to tell us about it—to be autistic means: having heightened sensory experiences (i.e., craving some while avoiding other sensory experiences); being confused (sometimes to the point of being terrified) with unpredictable aspects of the world, and actively seeking predicable patterns in the world; having a strong need to engage in a limited number of activities and/or learn about a limited number of topics to the exclusion of almost everything else; and needing to share one's experiences and knowledge about these things and, if this need cannot be met in relationships with others, inventing imaginary friends who "understand" them, or by just talking and listening to themselves. To be autistic means knowing (or feeling) that one is different and wanting to be acknowledged as such in a respectful way. Being autistic means not wishing to be "normal" but wanting to be socially accepted; it means wanting to "fit better" (i.e., to be in a greater control of one's thoughts and actions, so that one can use one's abilities and skills to perform better in society).

Who I am: Teodor's perspective

Now back to Teodor. We know how others—his family members, school staff and the psychiatrist—see him. And we know how he performs on psychometric tests and in psychological interviews. In the clinical interview, we began to hear Teodor speak for himself. In this chapter, we will continue to get to know Teodor more personally. We will learn about Teodor and his world from his own perspective through (1) casual conversation, (2) correspondence with Ljiljana, and (3) his autobiographical writings. Although still a young teenager, we will see clear echoes of the previous section in many of the things Teodor has to say about himself and his life.

"I'm a bus:" Teodor in casual conversation

Before beginning the clinical interview, conducted over three separate sessions, Teodor and Ljiljana had small conversations (Teodor was twelve at the time). Ljiljana asked Teodor to share some good and bad news about things that happened since they last met. Here are three examples of Teodor's good news. The first is about a trip:

Teodor: Yesterday, I went to Newmarket with buses—

Ljiljana: With whom?

Teodor: With my grandmother.

Ljiljana: And what did you do in Newmarket?

Teodor: Like—I waited for the other bus, a bus that I was gonna take, but I couldn't [a few months ago, when he last went to Newmarket, but missed this particular bus], so I took it now—when a—a bus that I've never taken, um, I don't mean a specific bus for a departure time but a bus that with the whole route I haven't been with.

Ljiljana: Um-hm, and—what did you do—you just took the bus and got home?

Teodor: I took the B bus, um, the one that goes on Yonge C, I mean that goes on the bus route that you take, but at Yonge and Bernard—there where the C bus turns around—the B bus continues to Newmarket—I took that one and—but she had to wake me up early in the morning.

Ljiljana: How early?

Teodor: Like, at seven o'clock—because that bus from Newmarket that we switched to—the last is at 8:30 and other in the afternoon when it's very hot—and—and there are some other buses that go where that bus goes, and—but they are not that bus, they go, like—that bus goes through King City and Maple, but that bus goes only along Highway 400.

Ljiljana: So when you got to Newmarket, you transferred to another bus and you came home?

Teodor: No, um, I went to Yorkdale, and then—with that bus I—I, like, copied the bus platform, like "platform number 3"—what bus is there—but not all because—like, my—I am afraid—I was afraid my grandmother was bored waiting.

Ljiljana: How long did it take?

Teodor: Approximately five minutes.

Ljiljana: Oh, OK.

Teodor: And, then we took the subway to Wilson, then a bus to York Mills, then subway to Finch, and the C bus—the one that you took—to Yonge and 16th Avenue and walked home.

Ljiljana: OK, and what time did you get home?

Teodor: Approximately eleven o'clock.

Ljiljana: In the morning?

Teodor: Yeah.

Ljiljana: All right. So how long was your trip?

Teodor: So, like—four hours.

The second good news is from school:

Teodor: Kevin [Teodor's best friend] and Victor [Teodor's second best friend] weren't working to help the caretakers anymore, and—like, Victor always hurries up to get a chair that he knows I like, and he barely gives it to me except if I leave and he says, "Teodor, I'm sorry, come on, you can get the chair." But, like, if I say, "Victor, can I please have it for today?"—"Nooo." [Imitates Victor's voice.]

Ljiljana: Um-hm. And so what's the good news?

Teodor: That I could get the chair.

Ljiljana: OK. [Laughs]

Teodor: And no annoying people.

Ljiljana: Sorry?

Teodor: No annoying people.

Ljiljana: What does that mean?

Teodor: Because, like, Victor annoys me and, like, I made a schedule for me—like, a bus schedule—like, I'm a bus and, like, I say, at room 120 in my school—I stop there on request. Like, at TTC it means—"on request"—when you pull the bell. But, like, "on request"—I stop there if, like, people annoy me very bad in the caretaker's office, or if, like, I say, "If you do that, I'm gonna leave," and someone says, "Leave!" [in angry voice]—that's a request too.

Ljiljana: Um-hm, and what do you do when you stop?

Teodor: I go there, like, when I eat in the caretaker's office, it means I stop in the caretaker's office. So I'm like a bus.

Ljiljana: I see, hmm—interesting. [Teodor: Yeah.] So you are playing bus in school?

Teodor: Only when I go from the playground to my class—I count it as a bus for my schedule, but I'm not playing bus like other buses, like, let's say in school I stop working and I play bus through the school—no, I play bus only when my schedule says, and that's at recess and lunch.

The third good news is from a visit to family friends:

Teodor: Yesterday, I went to visit some of my friends, and they... And they brought me some [bus] transfers!

Ljiljana: And [where] are these transfers from?

Teodor: From route 49. And, like, I had to ask them, because, like, they went with 49 but the transfer was a Kipling transfer, and where it said Kipling South, there was a circle, and that means it's route 44. But, like, I understand that Kipling—when it arrived—it switched in route 44. When we [Teodor and Ljiljana] went with route 49—that happened then, like, "How come? Now it's route 44?" Because it has transfers from 49—not from 44. That's when *we* went.

Ljiljana: And when did we go?

Teodor: Last—no—in 1998, in day 234 of the year.

Ljiljana: Are you joking?

Teodor: No. Like the year has 365 days; we went in day 234.

Ljiljana: How do you know?

Teodor: I see the picture of the transfer.

Now consider three examples of Teodor's bad news. Teodor pointed out that there were *two* bad news items in the following example, one about another person, and one about him.

Teodor: Yesterday—my mother was gonna go shopping today, and as soon as we were going from your house, I mean, she was picking me up from Ontario Science Centre, we were gonna go to the Sick Kids' Hospital because John, a baby who lives in Peterborough, like—at his birthday—you know a balloon—when it's tied, it has a rope like that [shows with his hand] that you hold it with...and that rope went into his eye, and they need to consult his eyes because maybe his eye—because it's possible that he'll lose an eye, and we want to go see him... That's one [bad news], and second, we were gonna go today and she was talking on the phone, my mother... And, like, my mother was talking and Maria, his mother, she was saying, "Come whenever you want," and my mother wants to come Monday. And I was saying, "Noooo, tomorrow," because this week—when I could have taken TTC trips, I didn't at all, and I was very bored of it, I was—like, my brain was saying, No, I just have to go today, but my mother planned to go Monday. And, like, she hurt my feelings.

Ljiljana: And what are you bored from?

Teodor: From not taking TTC trips.

Ljiljana: All right. And then what's going to happen—when are you going to see—

Teodor: On Monday—tomorrow.

Ljiljana: On Monday. All right. So how do you feel now?

Teodor: A little bit better because we were gonna come back in the evening and I wanted to go with my mother to Oakville or to Oshawa when we come back—to take trips. And I said, like, "Okay, then if we go Monday can we go to other towns?" "Yes, but not too far"—like, to Oshawa, so, like, that's a little bit better.

Another item of bad news is again about a trip:

Teodor: I was planning to go on another way, I was planning this way [draws a line in the air], like, no—she [the grandmother] wouldn't like that way.

Ljiljana: Why not?

Teodor: Because it's too much to walk or too many buses. I had to switch it because I didn't want to make her feel sad.

Ljiljana: Oh, so did she tell you that she didn't—?

Teodor: I ask her, "Is that okay?" and she said, "Not quite," and then I switched it.

Sometimes Teodor also wants to share some funny news. Here is an example:

Teodor: And guess what I did that's funny? I had, like, three cars, but two of them are buses that light up.

Ljiljana: Where did you have them?

Teodor: In my bag. Remember when we went on TTC trips that I had a bag through my neck like that? [Shows how he puts the bag.] In that bag that—that Nick bought me for Christmas—um—[sniffs]—like, I had those cars, and like, when I—we were watching the DVD, and I wanted to get something, I couldn't see because Anna turned all the lights off. And—um—like, that bus lights up very good, so I used it as a lantern and they could see [sniffs].

Ljiljana: And that's funny?

Teodor: Yeah... When I came, I said "I'm not Teodor—look who I am." [Points to his chest as if the police badge is there.] And, and then "Ahhhh!" [Imitates the girls' reaction.]

Before moving on, it is worth emphasizing that these conversation examples are typical of conversations with Teodor. Most of the time Teodor talks about his trips, transfers, or transit games; occasionally, other topics, usually involving friends, become a subject for conversation.

Commentary

From these conversations we get quite a different first-hand impression of Teodor as a person and his unique way of being than we do from previous perspectives, even from his clinical interviews. By listening to *what* he talks about, and *how*, we learned about Teodor's emotions—his happiness, sadness, boredom, fear, concern, and annoyance—his needs and interests, his thinking style, his memory, and his language and conversation skills in a real-life context. And, more importantly, we got a sense of how all these skills and processes combine to shape the person Teodor is. We also now better understand some of the things Teodor's family members talked about such as the "TTC stuff" and "hobby with trips," "not so good" interaction with children, and caring behavior towards others.

Teodor's happiest moments seem to be related to public transit. He is happy when he goes on bus and train trips, and unhappy when they have to be postponed, or shortened. Teodor's feelings are hurt when he does not take a trip when he wants to take one. Teodor can even be "bored from not taking trips." When Teodor wants to go on a trip, it is more than just wanting—it seems to be a matter of "having to"—as he said, "My brain was saying, No, I just have to go today." Teodor is also happy when he gets bus transfers from other people from the rides they took.

We saw some examples of Teodor's "taking care" and being sensitive to other people's problems, about which we heard from his mother and grandmother. We saw that Teodor is "afraid" that his grandmother would get "bored waiting" when they go on trips together, and she waits in the station while he copies the TTC information he needs. However, from the first conversation example (the first good news), it is not clear whether this emotion is a case of fear of not going on trips with his grandmother again (if she is bored too much), or a genuine care for his grandmother. The first "bad news"—in which he tells us how he changed his original plan after he asked his grandmother whether she liked his plan—seems to clarify this point by showing that he does care about his grandmother. He consulted his grandmother when planning his trip, by asking her about each route he wanted to take, asking "Is that okay?" He also seems to understand that his grandmother would have gone on the long trip he had planned, but that she would have been sad on it, and he preferred to be a little bit sad himself (for having to shorten the trip), rather than have her be sad. Finally, by sharing as bad news the accident involving a baby that he knows, Teodor also presented himself as a person concerned for people outside his family.

From these conversations, we also learned more about Teodor's interaction with his peers (and lack of it), which he spoke about in his clinical interview and which his family members also mentioned. First, we heard more about the way Teodor spends school recess away from his friends; during this time he plays alone—his transportation games such as pretending to be a bus and stopping "on request" and according to his schedule. We also saw that Teodor feels that some children (in school) "annoy" him, for example, when they sit on his favorite chair.[121] Finally, we learned that when Teodor goes with his family to visit their friends, he enjoys playing with children younger than himself; he likes to pretend to be a policeman and "scare" them.

We also got a sense of Teodor's communication skills and some of his speech characteristics. It seems that Teodor has an awareness that others do not know a lot about the intricate "TTC stuff" and he takes his time to explain what things mean. And he seems to enjoy doing it. For example, he provided details necessary to understand his trip to Newmarket, and what "on request" in the TTC means. We also learned about Teodor's unique speech pattern, which includes a lot of repetitions, direct quotes, and imitations of others' voices.

Finally, these conversations highlight the specific characteristics of Teodor's trips. Teodor does not take trips in order to visit particular places; rather, trips are carried out with a particular bus or train route in mind. For example, he spoke about going on a trip with a "bus that [he has] never taken." We have also seen that going on a trip means changing (and transferring) a lot of buses and trains, which requires a lot of time, both waiting and traveling. The Newmarket trip involved six different buses and subways and took around four hours while the "regular" trip from Teodor's home to Newmarket would take under half an hour, including waiting time. From Teodor's mention of trips to Toronto, Oakville, New,market and Oshawa, we see that his trips cover a large area—more than 3000 square kilometres during a two-week period. We also see that Teodor went on these trips with all of his family members, except for his grandfather, who "walks too slowly" to accompany him. Teodor plans his trips with a lot of care and with a lot of knowledge about different aspects of public transit systems. This knowledge includes schedules, timetables, routes, platforms, and the approximate length of a "trip" from one place to the other. Planning these trips requires using and coordinating many skills needed to orient in space and to estimate and calculate time. Finally, we got a glimpse into Teodor's vast knowledge about the transfers in his collection, including details about the individual transfers that he collected a few years ago. In addition, we learned that when he gets a transfer from somebody, Teodor needs to ask about exactly where the person got it, and the exact destination the person traveled to, because the same transfer can be used on buses with the same number but which have different start and end points. For example, some buses make a "short-turn," or go on a longer route than usual or change routes during the rush hours.[122] So, it is not the transfer in itself that is of central interest to Teodor, but the information associated with it; it loses its value if he does not know how the transfer was used.

"I can one day play with people at school both recesses": Teodor, in correspondence

Teodor occasionally writes to Ljiljana. He sends her e-mails, letters and postcards. He seems to like corresponding. When he was ten years old, after he sent two e-mails to Ljiljana to which she did not reply immediately, he wrote this message:

> Hi, my friend
>
> Today, I learned how to do math, concentrating a lot, making only a few small mistakes.
> I can one day play with people at school both reccecess [sic].
> How was your first day in school?[123]
> PLEASE WRITE ME AN E-MAIL BACK, BECAUSE I'M TIRED OF NOT GETTING ANY BACK.
>
> Your friend,
>
> Teodor
>
> September 13, 1999

Sometimes he likes to share his happy or sad experiences. Here are two such e-mail messages, also written when he was ten:

> DEAR LILLIANA,
>
> ON THURSDAY, A BOY NAMED SAM SAID "HI, Teodor." AND I SAID "HI" ALMOST LIKE HE SAID. MANY PEOPLE IN MY CLASS LIKE WHEN I SPEAK IN THEIR VOICE
>
> ...
>
> Teodor
>
> April 18, 1999

> Hi my friend,
>
> ...Today I went with 2 buses in Mississauga, but I had to give a tra[n]sfer to the second bus. Me and my father both said: "I collect them." But the driver said both times no. I was almost, almost, almost crying and I tried very hard not to, but most of the time I cou[l]dn't stop...
>
> Teodor
>
> August 19, 1999

At other times, Teodor likes to share "a joke." Here is one such message, with a subject heading "A joke, on Friday," written when Teodor was ten years old:

> Hi my friend,
>
> Pay Attention!
>
> I took Bus # 3 north from York Central Hospital, northbound. It goes to a terminal at Yonge St./Bernard Ave. Bus # 1C goes from that terminal to a GO train station. That's in Richmond Hill. When I arrived with bus # 3 at the terminal at Yonge/Bernard Ave., I asked the driver "Excuse Me?, are you going back to York Central Hospital?" The driver said, "I am a 1C now."
>
> December 3, 1999

Here is another "joke message," with a subject heading "DO THEM AGAIN!, joke," written when Teodor was eleven:

> Hi, my friend
>
> JUST LOOK AT THIS JOKE:
> I WANT YOU TO DRAW ME 3 BUSES!
> But I just finished. DO THEM AGAIN!
>
> March 3, 2000

Sometimes Teodor sends a "joke letter" by regular mail. Here are the highlights from a letter that consists almost entirely of Ljiljana's comments to him and other children over a two-and-a-half-year period:

> GUYS! YOU ARE MAKING TOO MUCH NOISE! [Said to a group of children in the hallway outside the room in which the "mind game" group was playing approximately two and a half years earlier.]
>
> BUT YOU DON'T NEED TO CALL A TIMELINE, BECAUSE YOU ALREADY HAVE A TIMETABLE. [Said to him approximately two years earlier.]

TEODOR? YEAH? WHY DON'T YOU WANNA GET OFF HERE AND TAKE THE BUS HERE[?]

WHY DO YOU WANNA GO ALL THE WAY TO SQUARE ONE? [A short dialog with him that took place approximately a year earlier.]

August 19, 1999

When Ljiljana asked Teodor why he sent her this letter, he replied that he wanted to remind her of the funny things she said; funny because of the way she said them. When Teodor goes on longer trips, he sends postcards. Here is a recent postcard, sent to Ljiljana when Teodor was twelve years old.

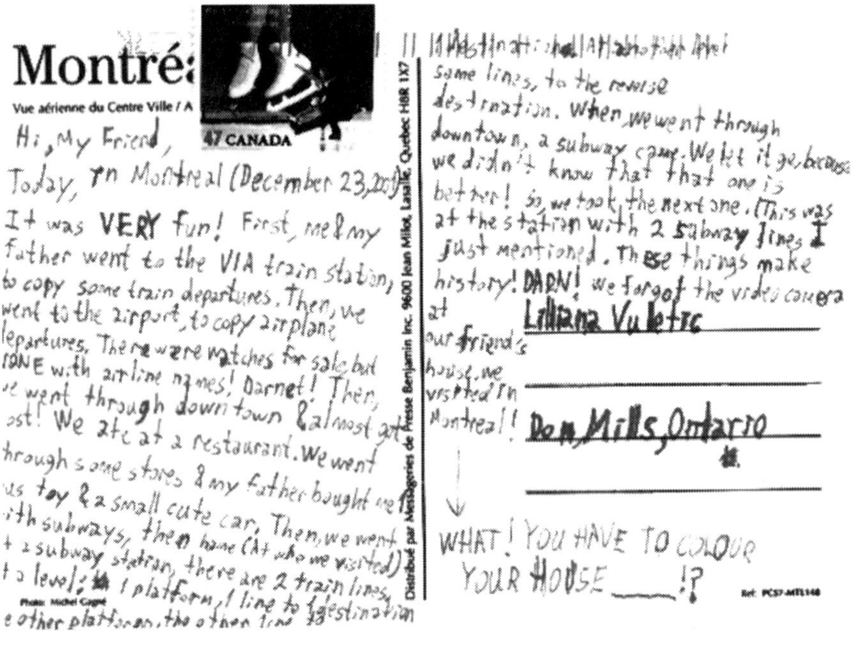

Figure 5.1: A postcard from a Montreal trip

Hi, My Friend,

Today, in Montreal[124] (December 23, 2001) it was VERY fun! First, me & my father went to the VIA train station, to copy some train departures. Then, we went to the airport, to copy airplane departures. There were watches for sale, but NONE with airline names! Darnet! Then, we went through downtown & almost got lost! We ate at a restaurant. We went through some stores & my

> father bought me 1 bus toy & a small cute car. Then, we went with subways, then home (At who we visited)[.] At a subway station, there are 2 train lines. At a level: 1 platform, 1 line to 1 destination[.] The other platform, the other line to 1 destination. At another level, same lines, to the reverse destination. When we went through downtown, a subway came. We let it go, because we didn't know that that one is better! So, we took the next one. (This was at the station with 2 subway lines I just mentioned.) These things make history! DARN! We forgot the video camera at our friend's house we visited in Montreal!
>
> WHAT! YOU HAVE TO COLOUR YOUR HOUSE............ [green]!?

This last sentence is one of the comments that Teodor was repeating for the past few months whenever he had a chance to. He originally made this comment while he was listening to his friend Kevin's description of his science project in which he had to make a "green house." Teodor interrupted him with the comment, "What! You have to colour your house green!?"—exclaimed with a great surprise in his voice and accompanied by a jerking movement of his whole body, his eyebrows lifted, and eyes wide open. Kevin and Ljiljana's reaction to it (i.e., laughing) inspired Teodor to transform it afterwards into many similar comments (which he considers to be jokes). For example, when he wanted to make Ljiljana laugh, he would say—in his regular voice, "I have a project on a bus." And then—in a very different voice, like Ljiljana's when she is very surprised, "What! You have to steal a bus from the bus department!?"

And here is what Teodor wrote on a postcard from a trip to Romania when he was eleven:

> Hi, my Friend
>
> I am in Bucharest, the capital of Romania. I visited lots of places in Bucharest & Romania and I went with lots of means of transportation, & even with a train to Sinaia, where I stayed 5 days. I feel good in Romania, but I don't have everything I need. We have another long train trip, and I think I will like it a lot.
>
> Your friend, Teodor Vuletic [Ljiljana's last name]
>
> August, 2000

When asked what he meant by "I don't have everything I need," Teodor said, "Internet," and explained that he *needed* to find information about public transit in Romania and other countries that he visited that summer.

Commentary

From this spontaneous e-mail and letter correspondence, we learned many important details about Teodor and his world, and got a better sense of Teodor as a person. Teodor's correspondence is usually about public transit and "fun with sounds." We see that, for Teodor, learning about public transit in new places he visits is fun. His goal for any trip or vacation is to take as many "means of transportations" as he can, and to collect as many tickets and transfers as possible. Consequently, giving a transfer to a bus driver (as is sometimes necessary when changing transit) and coming home from a trip without one is almost unbearable.

We now also have a much clearer picture of what Teodor's parents meant when they spoke of Teodor's fun with sounds, and what this means for Teodor. For Teodor, not only is verbally imitating voices fun, but also writing them in capital letters (perhaps his fun here is in "hearing" them while he is writing). We also learned that Teodor likes to share his "jokes" with others—his classmates and Ljiljana.

Most of Teodor's "jokes" are:

- just simple imitations of someone's voice (e.g., "HI," "DARN!")
- repetition/imitation of others' comments (e.g., "GUYS! YOU ARE MAKING TOO MUCH NOISE!") and of his own comments (e.g., "WHAT! YOU HAVE TO COLOUR YOUR HOUSE GREEN!?")
- their application to a new context (e.g., "These things make history!", "DO THEM AGAIN!")
- their playful distortion (e.g., "I have a project on a bus. WHAT! YOU HAVE TO STEAL A BUS FROM THE BUS DEPARTMENT!?").

In order to fully appreciate their humour, a reader needs to know the context in which these comments were made originally, as was clear from the example of the green house. Similarly, his "DO THEM AGAIN!" joke is only one of numerous playful alterations of his teacher's instruction to another student, previously described to Ljiljana.

Not everyone will find these jokes of Teodor's funny. In fact, we know that his family members dislike them. On the other hand, at least some of his classmates (and Ljiljana) like it when he "speak[s] in their voice." Teodor also has a more usual sense of humour—one that depends on appreciating non-literal meanings in speech, for example, when he told the story of a bus driver who announced, "I am a 1C now" instead of saying, "This bus is a 1C now." Finally, in his current repertoire of "funny things to repeat," Teodor uses others' voices from a few years ago, which suggests an extraordinary memory for sounds, intonations and short comments that have a high emotional charge and are rich in sound variations.

As regards his communication with others, Teodor enjoys both sending and receiving e-mail messages. He not only shares his jokes and school and trip experiences, but also shows an interest in others' experiences, for example, asking about Ljiljana's first day at school as a graduate student. Teodor also mentions short verbal exchanges he has had with other children (in which he imitates their voice). Interestingly, he "plans" to play with children at "both recesses" (indicating perhaps that he currently plays with children at one recess). However, this comment should be considered in light of Teodor and Ljiljana's earlier discussions about the use of recess time for play with children (which is something that Teodor needs to be constantly reminded of, to "think about" and make special plans for).

"I am a green transfer": Teodor's autobiographical writings

We now present four autobiographical pieces written by Teodor. The first was written for school back in 1998 and the other three more recently, at Ljiljana's request. For purposes of comparison, we also include an autobiographical essay written by Teodor's best friend, Kevin.

"TRANSFER BOY" (1998)

Teodor wrote this piece when he was nine years old, when his (then) new teacher asked him to write about himself through his hobbies, so as to introduce himself to a new class. This piece has three components (Figure 5.2). The first component is a drawing of a subway transfer with a face, coloured in green and labeled "transfer boy." The second component is the text, in which Teodor writes:

> I am a green Transfer. I eat a lot of other transfers. I look as a real transfer, but I have eyes. I am afraid of fire and seessiors [i.e., scissors].[125]

The third component answers a question written by Teodor's teacher: "What can you tell me about the TTC?" In reply, Teodor lists 26 subway stops in sequence:

> Kipling, Islington, Royal York, Old Mill, Jane, Runnymede, Keele, High park, Dundas west, Lansdowne, Dufferin, Ossington, *Christe* [*Christie*], Bathurst, *Spadana* [*Spadina*], St. George, Bay, Yonge, Sherbourne, Castle Frank, Broadview, Chester, Pape, Donlands, Greenwood, Coxwell [emphases added].

This partial list of subway names starts from one end of one of Toronto's subway lines and lists all subway stations of that line up to Coxwell, with only one sequencing mistake (High park should be after Keele) and no omissions. Since the list ends with a comma, and it does not list the end of the line, it seems reasonable to assume that Teodor did not finish his list for reasons other than lack of knowledge.[126] Note that Teodor made only two spelling mistakes on this list (the two words in italics)!

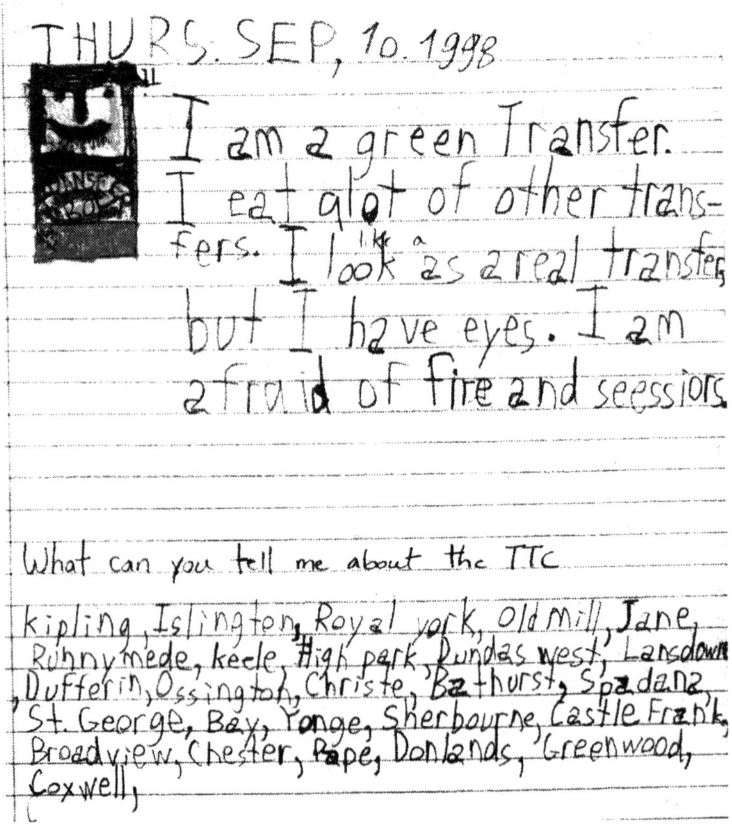

Figure 5.2: "I am a green transfer"

"WHY I LIKE TRANSFERS" (1999)

The second autobiographical piece was written by Teodor when asked why he likes transfers:

> I started collecting transfers in week 29, 1995. I thought They are very nice for me to collect, so I made a rule. I don't show my transfer If an adult dos'nt tell me to show my transfer. I like to collect transfers because I can use them as busies [buses] or as very nice things.
>
> Record of August 28, 1999

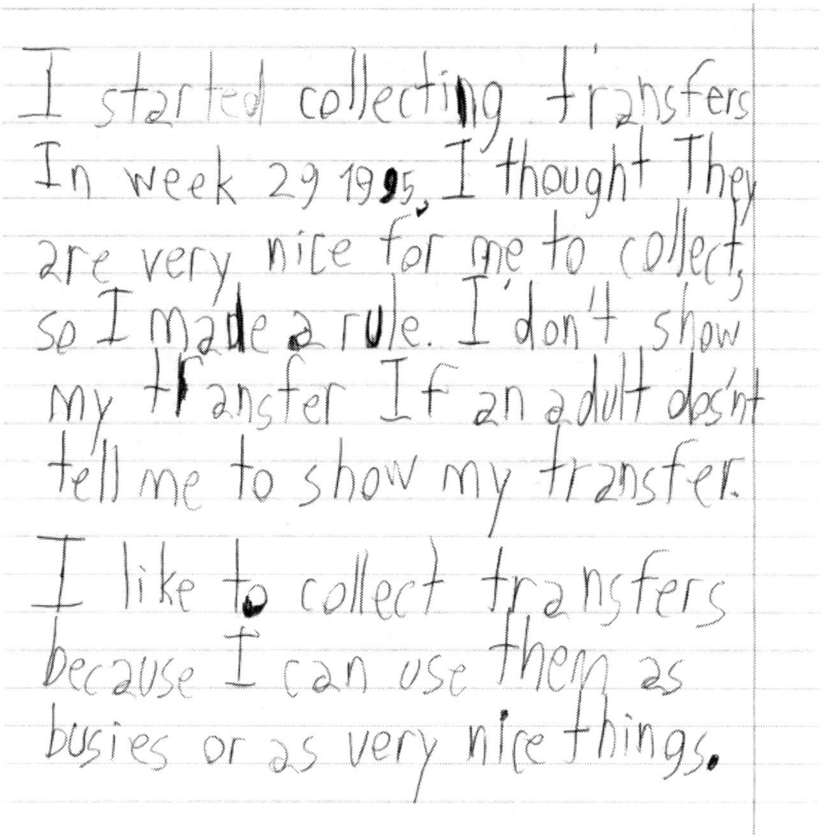
I started collecting transfers
In week 29 1995, I thought They
are very nice for me to collect,
so I made a rule. I don't show
my transfer If an adult doesn't
tell me to show my transfer.
I like to collect transfers
because I can use them as
busies or as very nice things.

Figure 5.3: "Why I like transfers"

"THE POEM ABOUT MYSELF" (2000)

Teodor often tells Ljiljana that he is very good at writing poems (something he also mentioned in the clinical interview), so she asked him to write one for her. This third autobiographical piece is what he wrote:

> I like transportation
>
> I like buses
>
> I like troleibuses
>
> I like streetcars

I like airplanes

I like subways

I like trains

"WHO I AM" (2001)

Finally, when asked to describe himself as he would to somebody who does not know him, Teodor wrote the following:

> **Who I Am**
> I am a person who knows and likes about different kinds of transportation. I collect lots, lots and lots of transfers from different buses, subways and streetcars, and trains. I also collect maps and schedules.
>
> I love having car toys and I make cars as buses by writing different destinations that I know and putting them on the cars. [Figure 5.4] I can also make cars as airplanes by putting wings on the cars and writing the company and the plane destination on a piece of paper and putting that piece of paper on the car.
>
> At school, during lunch recess, I help the caretakers in the school by washing desks in the classes. I love this job.
>
> I like drawing airplanes and building models. I also collect plane tickets and schedules. When I make my own plane schedule, I take information from the internet and I make my own schedules. I collect books with airplane pictures and in those books, there are pictures of airports showing the gate numbers and terminals (like a plan). I like watching movies, especially Home Alone, with airplanes and bad guys. The bad thing about that is that I hear, for example, "I'm gonna kill that kid," and I say, "I'm gonna kill you!" (This is a joke, of course!) and I get punished.
>
> I go on Sunday, with Lilliana to Ontario Science Centre. There, me and my friend play and learn!
>
> May 4, 2001

Before interpreting these autobiographical writings, consider also the essay Teodor wrote about his best friend, Kevin, as well as Kevin's essays about both himself and Teodor (written at the same time as Teodor's). We begin with Teodor's description of Kevin:

> **My Description of Kevin**
> Kevin is my best friend. His last name is Williams. Sometimes, he behaves bad to me, if he is in a bad mood, and accor[d]ing to what he does (hurts me, tells on me…), I punish him. He likes coming on bus trips with me. If he embarrasses me, I say, "1 trip cancelled!" This means, on 1 trip I take, he is cancelled to come with me (he doesn't come). He brings me my hobbies. He started to ask for extra transfers on each bus we take and unless I ask for one, I don't like

it. Since grade 7, he has lots of homework, so he barely plays with me. He comes with me to my best friend's house, and we go by bus by ourselves. In order for a trip to my friend's house to be cancelled, he has to do a VERY bad thing. He sits on escalator bars, when he knows he is not allowed to and I lift him up and put him down. If he does bad things, I call his parents to tell on him. He has a normal face and he is 12 years old. His birthday is on November 12.[127]

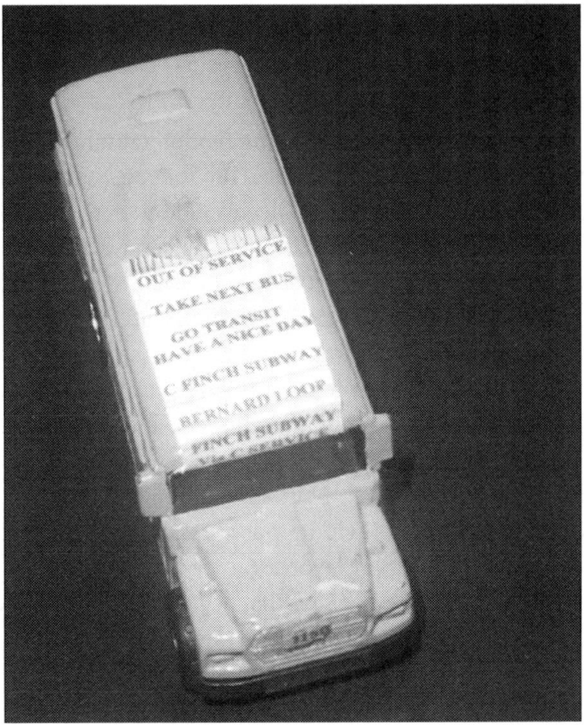

Figure 5.4: Teodor's toy bus. "The driver presses a button from inside the bus and the sign goes up or down to change the destination. The other destinations are on top of the bus and are not seen."

Here is what Kevin wrote about himself. Kevin has been diagnosed with a reading disability and with Attention Deficit Hyperactivity Disorder:

Who I Am

I am a kid. I am 12 year old. I am in grade 6. I like tools. I am very smart when it comes to fixing things. I like to learn. Math and science are the subject that I like the most. But I bet that I am the only kid in my school that knows a lots about tools. I know more then 200 kinds of tools. I have a

> best friend. [His] name is Mr. Teodor. So now I am going to talk about my favorite tv show, Pokemon and Alglomon.[128]

Finally, here is what Kevin wrote about Teodor:

> **My Friend**
> His name is Teodor. He is a 12 years old boy. He loves his transfers & he likes to take buses to get more transfers.

Commentary and reflections

Public transit is a reoccurring theme in all of Teodor's autobiographical writings, and even in his description of Kevin. In fact, Teodor consistently saw himself as a "transfer boy" over the four-year time span covered by these writings. In his most recent essay, "Who I Am," Teodor calls himself a person who "*knows and likes* about different kinds of transportation" and who collects transit-related objects and information. He describes one of the many ways of acquiring transit-related information—searching the Internet—and says how he uses this information to make his own transit schedules to play with.[129] He also writes about turning car toys into buses or airplanes and playing with them, and about drawing airplanes and making plane models.

However, Teodor also writes about three topics other than public transit: watching the movies, his "job" (helping out at school) and visits to the Ontario Science Centre. He tells us that his favorite movie is *Home Alone* because there are airplanes and bad guys in it. He also says that he particularly likes the way the bad guys in this movie say things and he likes to repeat what they say—in spite of sometimes being punished because members of his family do not like it when he does this. Finally, Teodor only mentions two other activities: his "job" as school caretaker's helper (saying only that he loves it) and his visits to the Ontario Science Centre (saying only that he goes there with his friends Kevin and Ljiljana, and that he plays and learns there).[130]

Surprisingly, some things are not found in Teodor's most recent essay. Only two people were mentioned (his best friend Kevin and Ljiljana) and then only in the last paragraph, perhaps added just for his audience—Ljiljana. School, too, is only mentioned in terms of his job as caretaker's helper, not in terms of his learning and/or his friendships, as one might expect in children his age.

Comparing Teodor's and his best friend's essays, we see both similarities and differences. Kevin writes about things he likes, just as Teodor does, and he writes in most detail about his main interest—tools. And just as Teodor writes about his favorite movie, Kevin writes about his favorite TV show. Kevin, too, mentions his best friend, but without providing any details. However, unlike Teodor, who starts his essay with the topic of most central interest to him—public transit—Kevin introduces himself in a most general way—as a "kid." Kevin then adds two more general things about himself, neither of which is even mentioned by Teodor: his age and school grade. Also, unlike Teodor, Kevin writes about school as it relates to learning (i.e., what he likes to learn the most). Surprisingly, Kevin mentions even fewer persons than Teodor—only his best friend, Teodor. Finally, although we find a greater variety of self-related themes (i.e., more breadth) in Kevin's account, Teodor's account has much richer descriptions of his "important" themes (i.e., more depth).

When we compare Teodor's and Kevin's descriptions of each other, we find interesting differences. Teodor mostly writes about Kevin in relationship with him and the TTC (i.e., what Kevin does when they are together, and how they get along) and only in the second introductory and the last two sentences tells about Kevin's other characteristics (i.e., his last name, age—including his birthday—and physical appearance). Interestingly, Teodor does not refer to these latter characteristics when describing himself. On the other hand, Kevin writes similarly about himself and his friend. He starts with general characteristics such as name and age, and considers the main interest in some detail.

Teodor's autobiographical writings also illustrate a number of his special skills and abilities mentioned earlier—and some new ones. For example, in his answer to the teacher's question about TTC, he displays some extraordinary abilities, including (1) recall of strange names, (2) spelling skills, and (3) spatial memory of the subway stations (learned not from studying a list of subway stations, but from taking subway rides). In Teodor's description of why he likes transfers, we again see his extraordinary visual memory for numbers; he remembers the exact week and year when he began to collect transfers, because this information is written on the transfers (recall Figure 1.2). Finally, although in all of Teodor's writings he shows very good writing skills, his "transfer boy" essay also illustrates his imaginative and literary skills.

What we learned about Teodor from himself

In this section, we will attempt to sketch a portrait of Teodor as a person, using the information he provided. We will do this from two different perspectives, using two different (although related) criteria of defining a person: by what one likes, and by what one remembers.

ONE IS WHAT ONE LIKES

When asked, Teodor said that the best way to describe a person is by describing what one likes. From this perspective, Teodor is best described as a *person who likes public transit*. In fact, he defines himself through public transit through all methods of inquiry used in this project, except for the paper and pencil Self-Perception Profile for Children (Harter 1985), which, as already pointed out, is a forced-choice instrument that constructs a limited range of profiles.

In the casual conversations with Ljiljana, Teodor presents himself as a person who really likes to take public transit trips, play public transit games, and learn about public transit. In his correspondence, he emphasizes his love for trips, his need for information about public transit, and his sadness when his needs are not met. In his autobiographical writings, Teodor portrays himself as a person who knows and likes things about public transit, collects items related to public transit, and plays public transit games. Even in the Self-Understanding Interview (Damon and Hart 1988), Teodor mostly characterizes himself as a person who knows and is smart about things about public transit. Finally, in the clinical interview based on Harter's Self-Perception Profile for Children, Teodor portrays himself as a person who is interested in and knows about public transit, collects things about public transit, plays public transit games, and cries when a public transit item (like a transit transfer) is ripped. Therefore, one might say that public transit constitutes Teodor's centre of personal gravity. Furthermore, Teodor often refers to himself as a "transportation [or TTC] expert," a "TTC person", and—in his poetic label in his school essay from a few years ago—a "transfer boy".

Teodor's need to have fun with sounds also seems to be at his centre of personal gravity. Even though this need was not as apparent as his interest in public transit, it could be recognized in most of the methods of inquiry we used. Through his correspondence in particular, Teodor clearly portrays himself as someone who seeks every opportunity to engage in repeating others' voices. There seem to be two aspects of this need: to hear the voices, and to share the fun with others—his classmates and Ljiljana—and to entertain them. Moreover, this need is so strong that Teodor is ready to accept negative consequences of engaging in this sort of fun. In the "Who I Am" essay, he mentions getting punished by his parents when he repeats his favorite lines from his favorite movie, *Home Alone*; in the clinical interview, he said that his friend Victor also punishes him by not sitting with him on the school bus after he calls him, "You little!", like he heard in the same movie.

Although Teodor talks about interests other than public transit and fun with sounds, he talks about different interests when we used different methods of inquiry. In both the Self-Understanding Interview (Damon and Hart 1988) and the Self-Perception Profile for Children (Harter 1985), Teodor talked explicitly about his interest in having friends and in doing well at school. In his most recent autobiographical essay, he writes about three new areas of interest: his caretaker's job, watching movies, and visiting the Ontario Science Centre. One way to account for these differences is that different lines of inquiry might have promoted mentioning different interests.

In the clinical interview, Teodor talked about wanting to have more friends. This may give the impression that Teodor really thinks about this issue or is even concerned with it. However, these comments were prompted by asking him to elaborate on his answer to the Self-Perception Profile for Children question about whether he has as many friends as he wants, or whether he would like to have a lot more friends. Nowhere else did Teodor even mention that he would like to have more friends. To the contrary, he prefers to play alone and avoids friends he has if they do not want to play his games. However, when asked to think about it, he perhaps realizes that it would be nice to play with children—if only they wanted to play by his rules—and he saw a possibility of that happening with some children that he does not yet know. Teodor's "plan" to play with children at both school recesses, mentioned in one of his e-mails, indicates that playing with others is not something he really needs. That Teodor's "plan" was not his idea (i.e., the expression of his need) is indicated by its vague formulation "I can one day play with people at school both recesses," and by the fact that Teodor only came up with this after he and Ljiljana had discussed the importance of having friends and playing with other children in school (as well as strategies that Teodor could use for this purpose). However, even though these responses were elicited, they do show that Teodor has *some* interest in playing with *some* children—under special conditions.

Interestingly, neither Teodor nor anyone else mentioned that—like Liane Holliday Willey—until recently, Teodor had *imaginary friends.*[131] In fact, he has one hundred of them and always refers to them as "my one hundred people." They "live" in his stomach and Teodor communicates with them through a special "language" that he invented and which is based on head and hand movements. Importantly, they love the same things that he loves: public transit and funny sounds—a fact that we take as an important indicator of the kinds of friends Teodor would really like to have.

Similarly, Teodor's interest in doing well at school was only mentioned when he was asked about school specifically, but he did not show a genuine interest in any of the school subjects. He only wants to get a good mark in school so that he can go on a trip as a reward. Still, since he often repeats the statements his family members make about it, he seems to understand that it is important to study for school.

Although Teodor mentioned his caretaker's "job" in his "Who I Am" essay and in the Self-Understanding Interview, he never said a lot about it. However, his statement that he loves it tells us that this job is important to him. Finally, only in the last paragraph of his autobiographical essay does Teodor mention visits to Ontario Science Centre with his friend and Ljiljana. And all he had to say about it was that he plays and learns there—which is really not indicative of a great interest.

For all the above reasons, we conclude that—although Teodor's interests in playing with other children, doing well at school, helping the caretakers in school, and visits to the Ontario Science Centre are not Teodor's main interests—these interests are the fringe of Teodor's personal gravity. This personal fringe can be conceived of as similar to Lev Vygotsky's (1934/1986) notion of the *zone of proximal development.* From this Vygotskian perspective, the most interesting area of a child's development is not to be found in what he or she can do right now, but rather in what he or she can do with the help of others.[132] Similarly, the most important area of Teodor's personal space may not be what Teodor is the most interested in now, but in what he *can* become more interested, with the help of others.

Finally, there are things that never came up in Teodor's accounts of himself. For example, interest in computer games, music, literature, science, fashion, TV shows, and other interests that children of his age would usually mention. Therefore, we see these areas of life as belonging to Teodor's most remote personal fringe, if they matter at all.

ONE IS WHAT ONE REMEMBERS

Some people say that the way we define ourselves is through our autobiographical narratives, which crucially depend on our memory (Freeman and Brockmeier 2001; Locke 1690/1997). Moreover, Mark Freeman and Jens Brockmeier (2001; also Taylor 1985, 1989) argue that the way we evaluate our past is inseparable from our conceptions of what a good life is, or should be. Clearly, Teodor organizes his autobiographical narratives[133] around public transit and funny things. When we apply this second criterion for defining a person, we obtain the same basic portrait of Teodor: he is a person who remembers information about public transit and "funny things." However, as these authors propose, these interests of Teodor have not only a psychological and aesthetic meaning (as the organizing force of his life, and a source of information about what a beautiful life is), but also an ethical dimension that informs Teodor about what constitutes a good life.

TEODOR'S PERSPECTIVE COMPARED TO OTHER FIRST-PERSON PERSPECTIVES

It is not surprising that we find both similarities and differences between Teodor's self-account and self-accounts of other autistic persons. However, because we are primarily interested in better understanding Teodor as a person (rather than in understanding autism per se), we have emphasized similarities.[134] From the reviewed autobiographical writings, it is clear that special interests are also at the personal centre of gravity of other autistic persons. Some have even had central interests similar to Teodor's. For example, Sean Barron too had a strong interest in buses—although school buses exclusively. Not only that, he too played in school by pretending to be a bus, and stopped at "bus stops:"

> Like each of the buses parked outside the school, I had my own route. The hallways were my roads, and I worked out my route and followed it precisely every single day. I needed to feel in control.
>
> Twice each day I followed my route... In the morning I went to my locker; then I began my route from there—walking to different set points in the halls and stopping at each one for a few seconds, the way a bus stops to pick up the kids. By the time I completed my trek it would be almost 8:50 A.M., when the tardy bell rang... During lunch I did the same thing. (Barron and Barron 2002, p.183)

In fact, many clinicians and researchers have reported an interest in public transits: buses, trains, and/or airplanes, and their schedules and transit maps (Asperger 1944/1991; Attwood 1998; Baron-Cohen 2000a; Hurlbutt and Chalmers 2002; Gillberg 1991, 2002; Tantam 1991; Wing 1981).

Teodor's second most central interest, to have fun with sounds (or the need to imitate sounds), is also commonly found in other autobiographical accounts of autistic individuals. Sean Barron also "loved to mimic certain TV commercials and programs to excess" and sometimes would "recite a whole scene word for word" (Barron and Barron 2002, p.180).[135]

Liane Holliday Willey's descriptions of her play with voice perhaps provide some insight into understanding Teodor's "fun with sounds." Not only did her play with voice provide Liane with pleasurable auditory experiences (through creating "new tones and pitch, different volumes and a myriad of rhythms" (1999, p.36), but also gave her some unique kinesthetic experiences (through the movements of different parts of her mouth when she uttered or wrote particular words: "I loved the way most words played on my tongue. I loved the way they caused different parts of my mouth to move" p.24). She specifically loved "words that tickled," "words that had smooth textures," and "words that warmed when [she] spoke them" (p.36). She also described enjoying the "feeling [her] voice left on [her] ear, the way it resonated in [her] throat and the sensation it created as it slipped past [her] lips" (p.36). When writing, she particularly looked for words that "looked, sounded and felt good" (p.36). She also "had to" mimic some voices because they were unpleasant and they "stung" her ears, but by mimicking them she "edited" them "into a medley [she] can appreciate and value" (p.36).

Could it be that Teodor had the same or similar need when he wrote some of his e-mails or letters to Ljiljana? Perhaps. We cannot answer this question now because Teodor cannot tell us yet what he finds to be "fun" in voices he loves to repeat, but we hope that he too will be able to shed more light on his experiences later, as his self-awareness develops further. Interestingly, neither is thirteen-year-old Luke Jackson very perceptive of his sensory experiences. For example, he writes of his love for lights:

> I do have a problem pulling my eyes from all glittery, shiny things. I have always liked lights and have loads in my room. I have a lava lamp, a disco ball, a UFO lamp and a magic mushroom... They are just hypnotic and soothing and such a wonderful escape from reality. (2002, p.69)

For Luke, some lights are "hypnotic and soothing," but he does not tell us why; how it feels to look at different lights, and where in his body it feels soothing (like a much older Liane Holliday Willey could tell us). And while Luke Jackson does notice and comment on some of the words in his book—"pub" ("I really don't like the sound of that word"; 2002, p.32) and "yats minging" ("does have a good sound to it"; p.100)—he provides no further details about what makes these words special.

However, although autobiographical accounts show that these intense interests are central to how autistic persons define they also show that themselves, these interests change over time and that childhood interests do not necessarily remain at their personal centre of gravity in adolescence or adulthood. For example, before Sean Barron became interested in school buses, he was fascinated with dead-end streets, but as a young adult, he stopped being interested in either of these and developed other, more mature interests such as the peace movement. Teodor too had had other intense interests (although not mentioned in any accounts—perhaps because they are the past now). Like Sean, he too loved dead-end streets, and like Jerry Goldsmith (Bemporad 1979), he too was fascinated with labels and prices in grocery stores. He was also intensely interested in dinosaurs and insects (in addition to buses and trains)—interests that lasted several years. Finally, although early interests often change over time (a fact also noticed by many clinicians; e.g., Attwood 1998; Gillberg 1991; Wing 1981, 2000), sometimes these interests develop into a career (as in the case of Temple Grandin).

On Teodor's personal fringe, we find an interest in having friends, although it seems that this means playing with other children according to his rules. Again, this is similar to what we find in other autobiographical accounts of autistic persons. For example, Donna Williams writes, "I knew how to create very simple games or adventures and sometimes allow others to participate, as long as it was *totally on my terms*" (1999a, p.29, emphasis added). This is what a "friend" meant to her:

> Sandra and I would play the same game every day. She'd laugh, I'd laugh, we'd laugh. We'd sit side by side and scream in each other's ear. It made me laugh because it tickled, and I really didn't care what it was that she was screaming. She was the first person to play my games. (p.26)[136]

It is interesting to consider Teodor's interest in having new friends (in spite of actively avoiding and rejecting invitations to play by his current friends, and saying that it is "boring" to play with his best friend Kevin)[137] in light of Donna's description. Taken together, they may indicate that when Teodor said that he wishes he had new friends, he meant friends who have similar interests and likes. Even though when Teodor was asked about why he considers Kevin his friend he mentioned having fun together, in his spontaneous statements about Kevin he never mentioned that; instead, he always complained about his "disturbing" him. The problem may be in the fact that Kevin cannot play the same game every day, and laugh at the same "joke" repeatedly. It is possible that Teodor expects a friend to do exactly that.

Moreover, as Teodor is getting older, the desire to find a friend who has similar interests might become even stronger. As Luke Jackson writes:

> I have now found that I occasionally meet someone who has the same interests as me. This is [a] fairly new experience and it's nice to have someone to talk to and spend time with. Don't get me wrong, I have always been a loner and don't mind at all that I am on my own, but it is nice to have a friend too. If you do have one, then try hard to keep them. I have spent years never talking to anyone at school and never wanting to, but now to have a friend is quite fun. (2002, pp.40–41)

On Teodor's personal fringe, we also find an interest in helping the caretakers. In his autobiographical essay, Teodor said that he loves his caretaker's helper "job." When asked more about it, he emphasized two aspects of this work: helping others and receiving recognition. We have seen in Damon and Hart's Self-

Understanding Interview that it is important to Teodor to feel helpful when he expressed a feeling of pride when he can help someone find information about public transit. Other autistic persons have written about it too. For example, Luke Jackson also writes, "I would like to think that I am helpful" (2002, p.13).

Finally, on Teodor's personal fringe, we also find an interest in visiting a place where he can "play and learn" (the Ontario Science Centre). Even though Teodor did not write much about what it is that he likes about this particular place, we find it interesting that another autistic person (from another part of the world) found this same place worth describing in her autobiographical book. Donna Williams, who at the time lived in England, in her visit to Toronto, also visited the Ontario Science Centre. In her book *Like Color to the Blind: Soul Searching and Soul Finding*, she writes:

> It was an amazing place with lots of things to look at and touch and listen to. There were loads of things to experience, experiment with, and learn from without having to interact with anyone. (1996b, p.258)

We cannot say for sure which of these features (sensory, social or both), if any, were the reason Teodor included visits to this place in his autobiography, but we could be more confident now that there may be a real reason for its inclusion, rather than just pleasing Ljiljana (who takes him there and for whom the essay was written), which was our original interpretation.

There were many other similarities between Teodor's and other first-person accounts. For example, like Teodor, other autistic persons write about using their sense of touch to understand things. Therese Jolliffe says, "I always feel that I can understand things better through my fingers" (Jolliffe *et al.* 1992, p.15). Sean Barron writes about the pleasure that sameness of texture gave him, "I loved the texture of chains. Each link looked the same and even felt the same as all the others" (Barron and Barron 2002, p.31). Perhaps some textures, like bumpy skin, could elicit the opposite feeling—the displeasure Teodor reported about his skin, which led him to conclude that he does not "look" good. Moreover, Sean Barron writes that "The feel of something that was not perfectly smooth was wrong to me" (p.15).

Finally, it is worth comparing Teodor's autobiographical portrait to the one created by thirteen-year-old Luke Jackson. We start by comparing Teodor's last autobiographical essay "Who I Am" to Luke's self-descriptions in his recent book *Freaks, Geeks and Asperger Syndrome: A User Guide to Adolescence* (2002). Luke first states his full name and describes his physical appearance in detail (i.e., his hair, eyes and stature), none of which were mentioned in Teodor's autobiographical essay. He then writes, "I would like to think that I am helpful and quite kind. I am very polite; I think that is very important" (p.13), and he later adds, "Most people say that I am very polite" (p.100). Interestingly, even though Teodor's family members, too, mentioned that Teodor is kind and polite, Teodor did not say this about himself. However, the notion of helpfulness is also found in Teodor's Damon and Hart interview.

Another point of difference is the awareness of their autism. Unlike Teodor, Luke Jackson writes, "One unusual thing about me is that I have what some people would call a disability but I call a gift—Asperger syndrome" (p.19). Interestingly, he learned this just a year earlier, when he was twelve—Teodor's age now. So when comparing these two accounts, remember that, unlike Teodor, Luke is actively trying to "find a balance" (p.30) between his unique needs and his need to fit in. In fact, he writes that one of the "Top tips to enhance your chance" in dating, is "Don't talk too much about your fascination" (p.175). This may explain why Luke first mentions his main interest, or as he likes to call it "specialist interest"—computers—only on page 22, and then only as an illustration for something others had said about him:

> Apparently I am very pedantic and speak slowly and monotonously. My sisters often tell me stuff like this! I am also told that I have problems with communication because I do not know when I am boring someone. I suppose this is true. I like to talk about computers and don't usually realize that others don't want to. Well actually I do, but when I am thinking about computers I am not thinking about anyone else. (p.22)

Interestingly, Luke also writes that he has "gone from thinking about computers ninety nine per cent of the time to only thinking about them ninety seven per cent of the time" (p.191). All this shows that he is "really trying not to stand out too much" (p.30)—at least in his writing about himself. He writes about what others think of him first, followed by his comments (e.g., "I suppose this is true"). We don't know how Luke used to describe himself before he knew that he is autistic and before he started making an effort to fit in. And we will have to wait and see what effect, if any, this knowledge will have on Teodor's autobiography, once he learns about his autism.

Luke seems to have incorporated many more others' descriptions of himself as his own than Teodor did. Another contributing factor is that Luke has six siblings—three of whom are older than him, while Teodor is the only child in the family. In fact, Luke often credits some of his current self-descriptions to his siblings (e.g., "My sisters often tell me stuff like this!").

Like Teodor, Luke describes in some detail his difficulties with team sports. However, while Teodor believes that he could do better if he only paid more attention to the rules, Luke writes that he hates sports and describes reasons other than fast-changing rules that Teodor called "additional" ("When I finally work out what I am meant to be doing or where I am meant to be running to, they have started doing something else" p.130)—lack of coordination, and confusing sensory stimuli coming from all directions that make the whole situation frightening.[138] And he also writes about negative social interaction experiences related to sports (such as those when no team wants him to play with them) —Teodor does not.

Luke also writes about negative social interactions with children at other times and situations: "All my life I have been bullied;" children "used to push and shove me and call me names and generally make my life miserable" (pp.135–6). He describes incidents of teasing and serious physical bullying involving pushing, pulling, kicking and punching (with one incident ending with his concussion). And even though bullying is a common experience of children with Asperger syndrome (Asperger 1944/1991; Attwood 1998; Bosch 1962/1970; Little 2001) Teodor never mentioned it (except for saying that some children like to sit on his favorite chair "on purpose"—but we saw that this was not a case of bullying because that chair is everyone's favorite chair).[139] And although from some of Teodor's descriptions of his interactions with other children there were some indications of teasing, Teodor seems not to pay attention to them—at least he does not talk about them as bothering him. Moreover, in the previous chapter, he described how he had fun with a boy who was trying to bully him on the school bus (see p.75); by not taking it seriously, and mimicking the boy exactly, he turned this bullying into a game.

So far we have compared some of Teodor's self-descriptions and experiences to those of other autistic persons, especially the experiences of Luke, who is Teodor's age. Although these accounts have many similarities and differences, we deliberately emphasized the similarities because they help us understand Teodor better. There is still no convincing scientific explanation for Teodor's "fun with sounds" that might be useful to him, his parents, and teachers. Only through the accounts of autistic persons who describe their experiences do we come to understand Teodor's experiences much better. For example, Liane Holliday Willey's (1999) descriptions of her play with voice opened up a whole new perspective on why Teodor found some utterances so much fun. They also provided a constructive direction toward which to steer this "bad habit" (about which we will say more in chapter 6).

TEODOR'S AND HIS FAMILY'S PERSPECTIVES COMPARED

When we compare Teodor's composite account of himself to his family's composite account of him, both describe Teodor's interest in public transit and having fun with sounds. However, unlike Teodor's typical descriptions of himself as someone who likes and knows a lot about public transit, none of his family members mentioned this interest in their initial descriptions of Teodor. Instead, they all mention Teodor's special interest only after they had talked about his connectedness, love and respect for family members. Thus, the main difference we find between these two perspectives seem to be one of emphasis. Teodor first and foremost perceives himself as a person who likes and knows a lot about public transit. For the family, on the other hand, Teodor is a good child, first and foremost. Furthermore, family members and Teodor differ in their evaluations of Teodor's goodness (i.e., behavior). While family members are unanimous in their belief that Teodor is a good, polite and disciplined child, Teodor does not seem to agree. We believe that this difference of opinion comes from the disproportionate family feedback emphasizing his misbehavior, which might have led Teodor to overlook his mostly good behavior. Finally, interacting with peers had an important place in both portraits, and in both there were indications that Teodor's social life needs to be improved. However, while all family members were explicit about this, Teodor only implies that this is the case; for example, he said that he is least proud of himself when he sometimes behaves "bad and lose[s] friends," or that "not many children like to play with me."

Reflections: Is there a middle way?

Ten or fifteen years ago, it seemed impossible to bridge subjective and objective perspectives on autism. In her analysis of autobiographical writings of autistic persons, Francesca Happé (1991), a notable researcher in the field, questioned the authenticity of first-person accounts because many have been written with the help of professional writers. According to her analysis, autistic people shift to new topics too quickly, repeat themselves,[140] use idiosyncratic language,[141] etc., and, in general, fail to talk about things that are of foremost interest to psychologists. In other words, she thinks that they are unable to consider the readers of their writings and cannot report reliably on their own subjective experiences. For example, Happé wrote the following about the autobiography of Temple Grandin:

> We get an important insight into Temple's view of autism in the following passage: "Geschwind...states that people with delayed left hemisphere growth have talents. If autism and dyslexia were prevented maybe the price would be turning potentially talented individuals into ones with mediocre talents"... Thus she seems to see autism not so much as a handicap but as an alternative cognitive style—and perhaps, if the social handicap is taken to be unimportant, this is a fair view. Interestingly, she begins the next paragraph, "Research with artificial intelligence may provide some insights...",

> confirming her lack of interest in the social aspects of the autistic handicap. (1991, p.212)

It is illuminating to read Temple Grandin's reaction to Francesca Happé's analysis. She wrote:

> I am very disturbed by the...chapter written by Francesca Happé... I was upset by this passage. "It is interesting, however, in conjunction with her (referring to me) evident lack of interest in her own and others' emotions—and it should serve as a warning to us that these autistic writers may not be interested in, or capable of, writing on those subjects about which we should most like to hear their views." I definitely have emotions... Happé questioned the accuracy of facts in my book because I had a co-author. This made me angry. I did not allow the co-author to distort facts and Happé questioned the facts that did not agree with her theory. (2000, para.1)

And she went on at great length to describe her emotional reactions in different situations—to prove that she has emotions, and that she can write about them. And this time she tried to have her readers in mind, as the following sentence indicates: "When Francesca Happé gets to this point in this article she will probably ask: 'You have still not discussed your emotional relationships with people'" (para.2).

Autobiographical writings of other autistic individuals also show that there is a growing sense of disappointment with scientific treatment of autism and persons with this condition. Some of these persons who wrote about their difficulties understanding others' intentions and emotions also notice that other people (including the experts) cannot understand their emotions either. The fact that anybody calls them mindblind makes them bitter: "They simply assumed that if they could not see my feelings, I could not feel them. I think this shows a serious lack of perspective taking!" (Sinclair 1992, p.297). Jim Sinclair wonders how

> people who understand the things I don't understand can't understand how anyone can possibly not understand them. (That sentence makes perfect sense. If you have to work a little bit to process it, you may get a slight taste of what it's like to have a language-processing problem.) (1992, p.298)

Jim is deeply disappointed with scientific overgeneralizations—particularly those that come from a lack of scientific interest in real-life experiences and actions of autistic persons. With a dose of sarcasm, he writes, "In May of 1989, I drove 1,200 miles to attend the 10th annual TEACCH[142] conference, where I learned that autistic people can't drive" (p.294). Others prefer just to make jokes about autism experts; they talk about them as belonging to two categories: high-functioning—those who understand autistic persons, and low-functioning—those who do not (Hurlbutt and Chalmers 2002). But, most of all, autistic persons are deeply saddened by this lack of understanding on the part of those who claim to understand. Jim Sinclair's poem (Moreno 1992) says it all:

> I built a bridge, and crossed it,
> but there was no one there to meet me on the other side.
>
> (p.98, reproduced with permission from Springer Verlag and Jim Sinclair)

However, Jim Sinclair also recognizes that the bridges need to be built on different foundations—and from two sides—and pleads for a different kind of "understanding"—without bias:

> [R]ecognize that we are equally alien to each other, that my ways of being are not merely damaged versions of yours. Question your assumptions... Work with me to build more bridges between us. (1992, p.302)

Fortunately, these autobiographical writings, and direct contacts with autistic persons at conferences and in other real-life contexts, seem to have had an impact on the way experts think about autism. Tony Attwood (1998), a clinician with years of experience with autistic persons, in his recent book on Asperger syndrome writes about the qualities of their personalities and abilities. According to Attwood, autistic persons are "honest, loyal, reliable, forthright and hav[e] a strong moral code and sense of justice. Their cognitive qualities include an exceptional memory, enthusiasm and knowledge about their special interest, an original way of thinking, good imagination and remarkable ability to think using pictures." He also writes that Asperger syndrome "is not a condition to be ashamed of, but one to express with pride" (p.179) and concludes that, "Our civilization would be extremely dull and sterile if we did not have and treasure people with Asperger's Syndrome" (p.185).

In an attempt to move from "arrogance to accommodation and acceptance," clinicians Tony Attwood and Carol Gray (the inventor of Social Stories (1998) as a way of teaching autistic persons social skills) decided to take a radical step and move from talk of "diagnosis" to talk of "discovery." In other words, they "transformed" the DSM diagnostic criteria for Asperger's Disorder into "Discovery criteria for aspie" (a "user-friendly" label for persons with Asperger syndrome). As Gray and Attwood write, "Unlike *diagnosis*, the term *discovery* often refers to the identification of a person's strengths or talents. Actors are discovered.

Artists and musicians are discovered. A great friend is discovered" (1999, para. 3, emphases added).

From this perspective, many characteristics of aspies' social interaction are seen as qualitatively advantageous (e.g., regarding others at "face value", speaking one's mind irrespective of social context, and avoidance of "ritualistic small talk" and superficial conversation). Similarly, aspies' language (termed "Aspergerese") is portrayed as full of positive features (e.g., conversation without hidden agendas, advanced vocabulary and fascination with word-based humour). Gray and Attwood also recognize many positive aspects of aspies' cognition (such as preference for detail and exceptional memory for details, encyclopedic knowledge of some topics, originality, unbiased decisions, pereverance and persistence of thought). Some of the other positive features of aspies, according to Gray and Attwood, include acute senses, skills in individual sports and games (e.g. swimming, bowling), and an increased probability of continuing education after high school.

Even Baron-Cohen (2000a) followed suit in his paper entitled *Is Asperger syndrome/high-functioning autism necessarily a disability?* In it, he argued that for persons with Asperger syndrome, or high-functioning autism, the term *difference* may be "more neutral, value-free, and fairer" than the terms "impairment," "deficiency," or "disability." Instead, he proposed that Asperger syndrome is "better characterized as a *different* cognitive style" (emphasis in original) (p.489), specifically, a style that is "object-focused" and not "people-focused." He listed 12 "behavioural features" that he considered characteristic of persons with Asperger syndrome or high-functioning autism. They include characteristics such as having strong and persistent interests; being very accurate at perceiving details; noticing and recalling things that other people do not; being fascinated by patterned material; and being fascinated by systems.

This recent shift in perspective represents a huge step forward in the science of autism. Fifteen years earlier Baron-Cohen (1995, p.1) proposed that autistic persons were best described as "mindblind"! or "blind to things like thought, beliefs, knowledge, desires, and intentions"! He warned that "We need to be careful about concluding that autism involves mindblindness and nothing else. Our suggestion here is that autism involves mindblindness as a core deficit, but that other deficits may co-occur" (1995, p.137). The question now is whether his article represents a new bridge between first-person (subjective) and third-person (objective, or scientific) perspectives. We hope so, but do have some doubts.

In his article, Simon Baron-Cohen (2000a) does write about positive "behavioural features" of persons with Asperger syndrome (or high-functioning autism)—but his data is taken solely from studies in experimental psychology. He cites no case nor clinical studies, nor does he refer to any autobiographical accounts. We cannot but think that for Baron-Cohen spoken or written accounts of autism do not count as evidence, unless generated under experimental conditions in the laboratory. So unfortunately it looks to us as if there are still strong barriers between the subjective and objective perspectives, and that more time needs to pass before these barriers are taken away. Even so, his more recent work shows that he has gone beyond considering autism merely in terms of deficits and has begun to explore some of the remarkable and positive strengths of autistic persons (Baron-Cohen 2000b; O'Riordan *et al.* 2001; Plaisted, O'Riordan and Baron-Cohen 1998; Wheelwright and Baron-Cohen 2001). We think that this drastic shift was inevitable once he got to know the autistic persons, like those he mentioned in the acknowledgements of his paper: Bridget Lindley, David Andrews, Liane Holliday Willey, Chris Wilson, Temple Grandin and (his own PhD student) Therese Jolliffe (all of whom he thanks "for discussion of these ideas" and credits David Andrews "for having introduced this topic at an early point" p.486). It is, therefore, refreshing to see that Baron-Cohen does engage autistic persons as persons, no longer just as experimental subjects.

However, although this recent emphasis among professionals on the positive aspects of autism and difference as opposed to disability seems a huge step forward for the scientific study of autism, when we consider the history—it is not. Ironically, in his original paper, Hans Asperger wrote, "We find numerous autistic individuals among distinguished scientists. The contact disturbance which gives rise to helplessness in the matters of practical life is typical of the absent-minded professor, and has made him immortal in jokes and cartoons" (1944/1991, p.74). Unfortunately, in her seminal 1981 paper, Lorna Wing disagreed with Asperger on this point. Instead, she maintained that autistic persons are not capable of original achievements and that they have only rote knowledge in their areas of interest. She proposed that autistic persons are best characterized by the "triad of impairments," adding impaired imagination to Asperger's core deficits of impaired social interaction and communication. Sadly, this new framing coloured all the scientific and clinical work on autism and Asperger syndrome until very recently.

Although said in a different context (i.e., with regard to the diagnosis of autism), thirteen-year-old Luke Jackson's recommendation seems to apply here too: "The answer to this is that doctors need to learn in more detail about the Asperger Syndrome and autism and listen to those of us who actually live with it" (2002, p.27). Had they, it might have saved us some valuable time and the hurt feelings of those affected (see http://isnt.autistics.org).

6

Conclusion

Where Do We Go From Here?

In this book, we set out to deepen our understanding of an unusual boy by integrating information from many different biographical and scientific perspectives on his life. We particularly attempted to understand what it is like to be an autistic child by exploring how Teodor perceives himself as a person. We discovered that Teodor's main interests, needs and self-perceptions have not changed for quite a long time (for about eight years). But we have also seen a recent emergence of some new interests—particularly social ones, including an interest in having friends, and in what others say about him. Based on what we learned from clinical and autistic persons' autobiographical reports, these are good predictive signs. But, unfortunately, the current state of scientific knowledge does not allow us to understand what brought about these budding changes, their relevance, predictive value, nor whether nor how to intervene. In this final chapter, we draw some general conclusions and suggest a few practical and theoretical implications of our endeavor.

Teodor as a person

We discovered that Teodor's personal centre of gravity revolves around two main interests: public transit and imitating sounds. We saw that public transit is central to Teodor's life according to all the investigative methods used, except for Harter's Self-Perception Profile for Children, whose forced-choice format did not allow this interest to be expressed. Descriptions by everyone who knows Teodor concur that this is his main interest. Another central interest of Teodor's is having "fun with sounds." In fact, this interest emerged as an important descriptor of Teodor in almost all the methods used (except, again, in Harter's Self-Perception Profile for Children) and in accounts of almost all individuals who know him (except his grandmother's). On Teodor's personal fringe, we also found interests in having friends, helping the caretaker, and visiting interesting places where he can "play and learn" with his friend Kevin. Importantly, these interests emerged only in Teodor's most recent autobiographical pieces and not in the accounts by others who know him, except for his mother's mention of his recent interest in girls.

From the perspective of adult autistic persons, the best way to help autistic children is by utilizing their special interests (or "obsessions"). Temple Grandin has written and lectured extensively about how these interests can be channeled into productive work (Grandin 1992, 1997; Grandin and Scariano 1986; see also Klin and Volkmar 2000). According to her, "Parents, teachers, and therapists should work *with* fixations and not against them" (Grandin and Scariano 1986, p.177, emphasis added). In saying this, she spoke from her own experience of developing a successful career out of her "fixations." Liane Holliday Willey (1999), too, wrote about her constructive use of imitating others' voices in drama classes.

Therefore, it is worth considering some ways of enriching Teodor's life and facilitating his growth through expanding his main interests in constructive and productive ways. For example, by engaging Teodor in science and literary projects related to public transit topics, he could learn about new aspects of the TTC. He might also be encouraged to interview TTC workers such as bus drivers, dispatchers and controllers for his school projects and learn about different jobs that he might consider pursuing in the future. He might also be helped to find a volunteer job with the TTC where he can be of real help and enjoy it. Or he might be introduced to the world of video games like *Train Dispatcher*—a video game entirely about figuring out train routes and schedules—in which Teodor can practice all skills necessary for making real bus and train schedules in a game context. Similarly, he might be encouraged to take drama classes and "perform" at "family theater" to develop his skills in voice imitation (as long as he can find performances that interest at least some of his family members).

Teodor's emerging interest in having friends is of particular importance since his friendships are something that most people who know him are concerned about. His description of his imaginary friends is an important indicator of what kind of friends he *really* needs—ones who appreciate the same things he does. Ideally, helping Teodor to find "like-minded souls" who share an interest in transportation would allow this interest to flourish in a way that also promotes social engagement. In the age of the Internet, it may not be a problem anymore. In fact, autistic individuals have already created a number of Internet-based support groups which allow them contact, support, and friendships within an autistic culture.[144] In the meantime, since Teodor seems to really enjoy playing simple games (outside the transportation themes) with younger children, facilitating more interactions with them is also important, because it is definitely a step forward from playing alone. Finally, fostering his friendship with Kevin around TTC trips, visiting the Ontario Science Centre and other "fun places," and playing board games that both of them enjoy seems to be the best direction.

Teodor mentioned several times that he likes to help others. He feels proud when he can help someone with TTC directions and he loves to help the caretakers in the school cafeteria. He likes to be recognized for his knowledge, skills and help. But Teodor has other interests that could be utilized in school-based "jobs." For example, Teodor loves labels—any kind of labels—postage stamps, street signs, and book labels. In fact, in Teodor's home library he labeled his books the same way as his school library does: mystery, adventure, fiction and so on. Each book also has the information sheet about the author of the book, book's title, the borrower of the book, the due date and the room number. As we have seen from autobiographical accounts of autistic persons, interest in labels is common in earlier years and some even study library science and work in libraries in adulthood. Assigning Teodor a job as a helper to a school librarian would both fulfill his need to feel helpful and recognized, and also further develop his library skills.

In his autobiographical essay, Teodor mentioned the Ontario Science Centre as a place where he goes with his friend Kevin. It is important that he mentioned his friend in this context. In fact, places like this, where many exhibits (or attractions) require interaction with others, or could be more fun when explored with others, are really important for Teodor. The more fun social experiences with children Teodor has, the more likely that he will develop a real need for interacting with other children and not just with adults.

Teodor's self-understanding

Some experts suggested that the life outcomes of autistic persons crucially depend on their self-awareness of their "peculiarities" and its capacity for motivating self-change (Bemporad 1979; Kanner 1971; Volkmar and Cohen 1985). For example, Fred Volkmar and Donald Cohen described a young autistic adult who had a "remarkably good outcome," and in their attempt to identify possible factors that led to it, pointed to his "strong desire to develop interpersonal relationships during adolescence" (1985, p.53) as one of the potentially crucial factors. Leo Kanner followed up 96 autistic children—only 11 of whom he characterized as doing well at that time—and says, "Unlike most other autistic children, [these 11 children] became uneasily aware of their peculiarities [during adolescence] and began to make a conscious effort to do something about them" (p.209). All these authors (Bemporad 1979; Kanner 1973; Volkmar and Cohen 1985) and some autistic persons in their autobiographies (e.g., Barron and Barron 2002; Grandin and Scariano 1986) noted that this awareness emerges during their adolescent years. Therefore, we were particularly interested in learning about Teodor's self-awareness.

Clearly, Teodor can appropriately characterize himself. His self-perceptions about his defining characteristics are corroborated by accounts of others who know him. According to the Damon and Hart interview, Teodor's self-perceptions are also age-appropriate. However, it is true that his self-evaluations of his "less important" characteristics—as assessed by Harter's Self-Perception Profile for Children—often differed from those of others who know him. But, as we suggested earlier, his self-perceptions are sometimes based on different, first-person evidence. We believe that anyone answering the Harter questionnaire from this perspective using this additional information would arrive at similar assessments of his competences. Importantly, we have also seen an emerging influence of others' opinions about him on his own self-characterizations.

Finally, we were particularly interested to find out whether Teodor perceives himself as being different from his peers in any important way. We found no evidence of that. However, his observation that other children have more friends than he does, and his realization that not many children want to play with him, may be the beginning of such awareness. Perhaps this initial awareness may lead him to ask himself the critical question "Why?" and to realize that he is different from other children. We will have to wait and see whether this happens, and how he conceives of this difference, if it does happen; specifically, whether and how it will affect his emerging interest in playing with other children or any other aspect of his life. Certainly, it is better to discuss what "different" means before Teodor starts feeling that there is something "wrong" with him. Autistic persons have repeatedly told us about the difficulties associated with the effort to change negative self-esteem; and the effects of remedying the negative consequences of the feeling of "wrongness," "badness," and inadequacy are always uncertain.

Having in mind clinical and autistic persons' observations, and the urging of autistic persons that autistic children be told of their difference, we might want to intervene right now and tell Teodor about his autism in the hope that it will lead to his "conscious effort to do something" about it (Kanner 1973, p.209). However, in order to do this, one should be absolutely sure that Teodor is ready for this learning—that the benefits will outweigh the costs. Learning prematurely about one's limitations might be terrifying and overwhelming, even when they are presented in as unthreatening a manner as possible.[145] In fact, it can sometimes even lead to clinical anxiety, depression and other psychological disorders (Klin and Volkmar 2000; Tantam 2000). But, how can one tell if Teodor is ready? And how can one know which road is better: to wait or to tell? And what is the best thing to say? What are the best coping strategies to teach? These are some of the questions we might hope a science of autism could answer.[146]

What a science of autism/Asperger syndrome should be

In this final section we highlight some components missing from the scientific study of autism and suggest how we might progress more quickly toward a better understanding of autism/Asperger syndrome.

By definition, scientific categories should be as precise as possible; however, there is currently little agreement about what exactly Asperger syndrome is, and how it differs, if at all, from Autistic Disorder. In our opinion, more cross-sectional (or snap-shot) studies using our current imprecisely defined categories are not going to be very helpful. We do not even find it surprising that, after more than six decades of studying autism (and after thousands of studies and books about autism have been published), we still do not know how autism develops (i.e., what characterizes autism at different developmental points), nor how to best intervene at different developmental levels.[147]

To understand autism, we need not just more effort, but a different kind of effort. The great Russian psychologist, Lev Vygotsky, was perhaps among the first scholars to realize that

> a child whose development is impeded by a defect[148] is not simply a child less developed than his peers but a child who has developed differently. A child in each stage of his development, in each of his phases, represent[s] a qualitative uniqueness, i.e., a specific organic and psychological structure; in precisely the same way, a handicapped child represents a qualitatively different, unique type of development... If a blind child achieves the same level of development as a normal child, then the child with a defect achieves this in another way, by another course, by other means; and, for the pedagogue, it is particularly important to know the uniqueness of the course along which he must lead the child. This uniqueness transforms the minus of the handicap into the plus of compensation. (Vygotsky, Rieber and Carton 1924/1993, p.30)

Several important implications for the study of autism result from adopting this perspective on the development of autistic persons.

Autism as a dynamic developmental process

In other words, autism is not manifested in the same way in all autistic persons, nor does it stay unchanged over time. Autism develops, but not as a linear process—autism is a process whose development depends on the dynamic interactions of a "totality" of "coexisting" factors (to use Kurt Lewin's terms; 1951) with mutual influences. As Annette Karmiloff-Smith has suggested, echoing Vygotsky more than half a century later, "The dynamics of development itself are the key to understanding developmental disorders" (1998, p.398).

From her first-person perspective, Donna Williams knows that, "'Autism' as an experience describes a very complex interplay between identity, personality, environment, experience and the equipment with which to integrate and make sense of that experience" (1998, p.9). In other words, autism is only one feature of autistic persons, whose development is influenced by all kinds of protective and risk factors. Some factors are specific to the child, including genetic, maturational, temperamental, sensory, attentional, cognitive, social, emotional, volitional, and psychiatric[149] characteristics. Other factors are specific to the parents, family, and sociocultural environment. These factors include the level of caregivers' understanding of the child's behaviors, the caregivers' goals and motivations, their level of hope and optimism, and their type and amount of involvement with the child, as well as many other psychological, psychiatric, sociological, and economic influences. And, in fact, without considering the influence of as many factors as possible, we are bound to end up with a superficial and/or wrong interpretation of the results of our studies.

Given the multitude of factors that can influence the development of autism and their dynamic reciprocal interactions over time, it is clear that the current research practice—studying an isolated aspect of autism (i.e., the dependent variable) and "controlling for" a minimal number of confounding factors (usually intelligence, language, sex, and/or age)—with a particular obsession for studying cognitive and language skills—is far from satisfactory. Given this approach, with its "ritualized" hypothesis testing and its narrow focus on "explained variance" (Richters 1997), it is not surprising that we still do not know which factors facilitate good or bad life outcomes for autistic persons, except for the two factors most controlled for: cognitive and language skills (Howlin *et al.* 2004). Interestingly, these two factors were found to be decisive for life outcomes more than three decades earlier (Rutter *et al.* 1967), but even then not for children without severe mental retardation. In 1978, Michael Rutter wondered, "The outcome for mildly retarded or normally intelligent autistic children is less easy to predict than the outcome for the more severely handicapped. Some do much better than expected and some do much worse. Why?" (1978, p.498).

A quarter-century later, we still cannot answer that question. In order to start answering it, and in order to understand the development of autism, a different approach is necessary. A *dynamic systems approach* (Fogel 1990, 1993; Granic and Hollenstein 2003; Thelen and Smith 1994)—one that emphasizes the mutual reciprocal interactions among the elements of a multidimensional system across different contexts and developmental time points, while remaining sensitive to narrative and autobiography (Lewis and Ferrari 2001)—comes the closest to the challenge.

The varied expression of autism in different contexts

As Donna Williams tells us "[Autism] can appear, disappear and reappear in varying degrees in different circumstances" (1998, p.9). In order to capture this diversity, we must study it in real-life situations. In other words, to advance our understanding of autism, we must move from studying "autistic subjects" in "strange contexts" to studying autistic persons in the real world. As the psychologist Uri Bronfenbrenner has argued for a quarter of a century (1979, 1989), studying autistic persons seems to require the method advocated earlier by Kurt Lewin that involves understanding the life space, the "person-in-context"—"the person and the psychological environment as it exists for him" (1951, p.57) and which includes needs, motivation, mood, goals, anxiety, and ideals. Studying autistic persons in naturalistic settings can help us understand them as persons—including their unique experience, their strengths and weaknesses, their needs and interests, and their understanding of different aspects of the world—including their and others' minds, their attention, emotions, language, or any other psychological processes and constructs that we might find worth studying. And, in fact, there is very little empirical data about the functioning of autistic persons in everyday situations (e.g., Hauck *et al.* 1995; Ruble and Scott 2002; Stone and Caro-Martinez 1990; Toomey and Adams 1995).

Autism as a personal characteristic

Autism is an aspect of particular persons—and persons are not passive entities; they are proactive and future-oriented. Persons are agents of their lives. This means that they play an active role in their own development; they have needs, desires, intentions, values and goals. As the psychologist Albert Bandura has suggested, "People are not just onlooking hosts of internal mechanisms orchestrated by environmental events. They are *agents* of experiences rather than simply undergoers of experiences. The sensory, motor, and cerebral systems are tools people use to accomplish the tasks and goals that give meaning, direction, and satisfaction to their lives" (2001, p.4). And this point applies to autistic people, too. Their autobiographies are the evidence of that. This point was also made by the philosopher Charles Taylor (1989), when he wrote that our identity is expressive of our being a certain sort of person, not merely of our biological or psychological characteristics. However, for the most part, studies of autism still mostly concern what characterizes autism and not persons who are autistic.

To study autism as an expression of persons, we need a different kind of approach. Many philosophers, psychologists and neurologists (Allport 1937, 1955; Bruner 1990, 1997, 2002; Cytowic 1993; Ferrari and Mahalingam 1998; Freeman 2001; Freeman and Brockmeier 2001; Gardner 1997, 2002; Harré 1983; Kelly 1955; Luria 1968, 1972, 1979; MacIntyre 1981; McAdams 1990, 1993, 1995; Oatley 1992; Polkinghorne 1988; Ricoeur 1987; Sacks 1987, 1996; Taylor 1989) suggest that a proper method for studying persons is self/narrative (or auto/biography). As neurologist Richard Cytowic (1993) writes—in a different, but related context of neurological illnesses—we need to understand "real people, their needs, their feelings, and *what their illnesses mean to them*" (p.12, emphasis added). However, the application of self/narrative to autistic persons is fairly recent, and there are not many studies of this kind (Cesaroni and Garber 1991; Hurlbutt and Chalmers 2002; Volkmar and Cohen 1985). In this book, we applied this approach in an effort to understand Teodor as a unique person. When considering the importance of narrative, we need to consider the narrative people make of their own lives, and this depends on their capacity for self-awareness.

Self-understanding of autistic persons

In this book, we placed a particular emphasis on Teodor's self-understanding[150] because such awareness is the first step towards agentic action, and towards the realization of one's possibilities. There are two reasons why self-understanding of autistic persons is an important issue from both theoretical and practical perspectives.

The importance of self-knowledge has been highlighted throughout the history of human thought starting perhaps with the famous ancient Greek dictum "know yourself." As William James suggested over a century ago, unlike other kinds of knowledge, self-knowledge has a special status among all other kinds of knowledge (including knowledge of others) in that it "is felt" with "warmth and intimacy" (James, 1890, p.298)—and therefore has self-motivating power (i.e., the potential to influence the change of the self). Interestingly, this aspect of self-knowledge is absent from some modern influential psychological conceptions, which emphasize the cognitive aspects of self, like Harter's "self-concept" (Harter

1998, 1999), but there are also exceptions, like the concept of "possible-selves" (Markus and Nurius 1986). But, as novelist Milan Kundera puts it, "'I think, therefore I am' is the statement of an intellectual who underrates toothaches" (1991, p.225).

As discussed earlier, self-awareness is also thought to play a crucial role in the successful life outcomes of autistic persons. However, it has often been claimed that autistic persons are severely deficient in their ability for self-understanding.[151] According to the Theory of Mind deficit hypothesis, autistic persons are severely deficient in their ability to understand themselves, read their own minds, self-reflect, produce self-report and so on (Baron-Cohen 1989a, b, c, 1995, 2000b; Baron-Cohen *et al.* 1985, 1986; Happé 2003). Surprisingly, this claim has not been derived from empirical studies or clinical reports of autistic people. Rather, it has been derived from the theory which posits that self-understanding parallels understanding of others (Premack and Woodruff 1978). Consequently, almost all "scientific evidence" about self-awareness of autistic persons was logically derived from studies of autistic persons' understanding of others' minds.[152] As reviewed, these ToM studies found that autistic persons have difficulties in understanding others' false beliefs, and from this it is inferred that they also must have difficulties understanding their own minds, including their own experiences.[153] Despite the lack of any solid evidence, this claim has been repeated over and over in the literature and at scientific conferences.[154]

Self-understanding has been explored extensively in developmental psychology and we know quite a lot about typically developing children's conceptions of themselves and how they develop (for reviews see Damon and Hart 1988; Harter 1998, 1999) and about development of their ability to self-reflect (for a review see Flavell 1999). However, surprisingly little is known about self-understanding of autistic children and about their ability to self-reflect. As we have seen, only two studies systematically explored autistic children's self-understanding (Capps *et al.* 1995; and Lee and Hobson 1998), and several studies investigated their understanding of specific aspects of self-knowing such as intentions (Phillips *et al.* 1995; Russell and Hill 2001) and desires (Tan and Harris 1991). The lack of knowledge in this area is particularly striking when compared to our knowledge about autistic children's understanding of others' minds (their false beliefs in particular, which has been reported in over one hundred journal articles and several books; for a recent review see Baron-Cohen 2001). Fortunately, several case studies fill this gap by reporting the first-person accounts of older autistic children (Cesaroni and Garber 1991; Volkmar, Klin, Schultz, Rubin, and Bronen 2000) and of autistic adults (Bemporad 1979;

Cesaroni and Garber 1991; Hurlbutt and Chalmers 2002; Volkmar and Cohen 1985). Even more fortunately, as we have seen, autistic persons have started publishing their autobiographies from which the interested reader can learn about their self-understanding.

Indeed, from the published autobiographies of autistic persons, we have seen that this kind of knowledge has led to all kinds of self-interventions and self-improvements. This is particularly true of the self-knowledge as acquired through the process of writing one's autobiography. As Donna Williams puts it, "A good biography is not once or twice removed, but direct and felt, experienced and, one hopes, comprehended too, to the core of one's being" (1998, p.9). And when this happens, it may lead to the dramatic transformations in personal identity about which Donna Williams and other autistic persons have told us.

This motivating characteristic of self-knowledge has important implications for interventions designed to remedy the lack of social understanding of autistic persons. It is possible that autistic persons' self-knowledge—which includes one's awareness of one's lack of social understanding—has to precede any teaching about others (including their minds) because it can motivate one for its genuine acquisition. Only after an autistic person becomes intrinsically motivated (i.e., self-motivated) to learn about others, will other-mediated interventions lead to a meaningful and useful knowledge. Without it, we believe, all Theory of Mind teaching and any other social skills training will lead to accumulation of yet another kind of rote and idle knowledge that cannot be used outside of the context in which it was learned (as some studies have already shown, e.g., Ozonoff and Miller 1995).

Rather, as psychologist Robert Sternberg (1997) has suggested, the most important determinant of one's life success may be knowing one's strengths and weaknesses, and finding ways to capitalize on the strengths while compensating or correcting the weaknesses. He calls this aspect of self-understanding "successful intelligence" and argues that the most successful among us are those who have found the best ways to exploit their patterns of strengths and weaknesses. Interestingly, this kind of intelligence (which is really self-knowledge) has never been studied in autistic persons, let alone "controlled" for studies of their life outcomes.

We have seen that Teodor, for example, has this kind of self-knowledge. He knows what he is good at, and engages in those activities. And he knows what he is not good at (e.g., sports) and avoids them. Moreover, he is also aware of his attentional problems when the TTC pictures come to his mind during the class, and is actively trying to control them, as did Sean Barron (Barron and Barron 2002). Indeed, from Sean Barron's and all other autistic persons' autobiographies, we heard about their conscious effort to overcome many of their autistic habits.

But this does not mean that a high level of self-understanding (nor a high level of understanding of others) is a *sine qua non* (i.e., the absolute prerequisite) of a fulfilling life. In fact, autistic persons—as all other persons—certainly must vary greatly in their capacity for self-understanding and self-control, and not all of them will be able to achieve the level of agency that is evident in some autistic persons' autobiographies. Our next point underlines the other side of self-control: others' control, or care.

Autism-in-relation

In 1944 Hans Asperger wrote, "[B]ehind the cool and objective interaction with Fritz and all similar children there needs to be *genuine care* and kindness if one want[s] to achieve anything at all" (1944/1991, p.48, emphasis added). We believe that genuine care, that is, acceptance, respect and compassion for a fellow person—who happens to be autistic—is the most important of all influences on the development and expression of autism. We mean this not only in terms of the care of parents and caregivers, but of everyone—classmates, teachers, co-workers, neighbors, fellow-passengers on the bus, policy makers, researchers and anyone else who comes in contact with autistic persons. Although we believe that autism does involve genetic factors that constitute an individual difference situated *within* an autistic person, it certainly develops *among* autistic and nonautistic persons situated in a particular cultural and historical milieu, and therefore can no longer be said to exist within the autistic person alone. To acknowledge our share in autism, we call it autism-in-relation. If we want to humanely understand what autism-in-relation is, we need to look beyond autistic persons' lives in isolation.

When we humanely understand autistic people as subjects, we act differently than when we objectively understand them as objects for science. Unlike our contact with objects, when we meet autistic persons, we not only partially determine that particular autistic person's moment of autism-in-relation—we are also responsible for future expressions of autism-in-relation. As philosopher Martin Buber has suggested, when we meet another person, we must begin by accepting that person, which means "being able to tell, or rather not to tell, but only to make it felt to the other person, that I accept him just as he is…accepting how he ever is in this moment, in this actuality of his" (1965, p.181–182). But then, if we really care, we go beyond accepting, and "confirm" the other, where:

> confirming means first of all, accepting the whole potentiality of the other…potentiality that is meant by him and it can now be developed, it can evolve, it can answer the reality of life. He can do more or less to this scope but I can, too, do something. (p.182)

For Martin Buber, this accepting and confirming attitude of a person toward the other person allows the other to grow, to unfold, and to become whatever one can. But "helping someone unfold should not be confused with concepts such as arrogance and humility" (p.84). We think this view applies to any relationship with autistic persons, too. When we suggest that we should be concerned with autism as what Buber calls "interhuman," we see it as our responsibility to make it possible for autistic persons to experience their relationships, not only as unthreatening but as desirable—growth-promoting. Emphasizing their lack of social understanding only shows our limitations in engaging different kinds of minds. Likewise, if we call them social failures, we must accept our share in that failure. We should allow our encounters with them to be mutually enjoyable and a learning experience, just letting them be—creative, productive, and different.

As for those of us who are students of autism (current and future scientists—researchers and theorists), we should engage in what Martin Buber calls a "genuine dialogue" and "make present which is possible" (1965, p.85).[155] We could start with welcoming the autistic other into our world—world of science—by letting them tell us their story, by asking them[156] and respecting their perspectives, and considering them equal partners in progressing toward our mutual goal—genuine understanding of autism—accepting autistic persons as co-investigators and co-researchers.[157]

The next step should be less difficult—integrating this new and authentic interhuman perspective into a unified view of autism-as-relation. Such an integration will move from the current impasse of the two monologic and mutually exclusive ways of understanding autism discussed in our book: scientific and autobiographical. We might then discover some pieces missing from our "pure scientific account" of autism and gain some insight into how to resolve the Autistic Disorder vs. Asperger syndrome dilemma. We might begin to appreciate the range and variety of ways of being autistic, from Kanner's autism to "normality" with just a "dash of autism." But perhaps—having a "theory of mind"—we should appreciate what it must be like to be called "mindblind" regardless of how accurately it describes the condition, and stop using that term. And we could educate those in everyday contact with these "anthropologists from Mars"[158] about meeting their unique needs, if they do not impinge on others' needs. A particular emphasis should be placed on autistic persons' need for *care—not cure.*

Indeed, this movement toward care (or "the interhuman") has already begun. We see Canadian scientist Laurent Mottron's statement of support for the autistic person Michelle Dawson's open letter to the Canadian Government, as the beginning of a genuine dialog. Laurent Mottron writes:

> What she [Michelle Dawson] says drastically changes all that we are used to thinking regarding autism, and our ideas about what help we can provide… I am grateful to her for having opened my eyes to the human and historical dimensions of autism, when I saw it only as a handicap with a scientific enigma added. (*NO AUTISTICS ALLOWED*, Comment from Dr Laurent Mottron, 2003, in Dawson 2003)

Indeed, Laurent Mottron has shown that Buber's "interhuman" is possible between scientists and autistic persons by acknowledging a personal human dimension to autism. We see this as radically different from listing autistic persons' attributes, as demonstrated in scientific studies, where autism is treated as "a handicap with a scientific enigma added" and autistic persons are "guinea-pigged" (Williams 1999b, p.38), and considered representative of a group defined by averages.

And yet, in spite of many long-standing criticisms about the very notion of the concepts of "average child" and "average environment" and the impossibility of making an inference from "an abstractly defined 'average child'" to "a certain child at a certain moment" (Lewin 1931/1935, p.37), group design studies are still considered a "must" in the field of autism. In such studies, which John Richters rightly calls studies "of variables over individuals" (1997, p.199), autistic persons have typically been reduced to their core deficits or—an increasingly popular variant—their core assets. This mechanistic emphasis on controllable variables has generated a vast amount of information about the "core" components of autism with no clear view of how to put all this information together—and with some important components still missing—into an account that captures what autism is and what it is like to be autistic. However, at least some researchers in the field of developmental disabilities have started to argue that group design studies are "inherently limited in their effectiveness for identifying characteristics of individuals with a syndrome" and that we must study "the pattern of performance of individuals" (Mervis and Robinson 1999, p.117; see also Mervis and Klein-Tasman 2004). We agree, and add that there is still more to persons than their performance, and that understanding autistic persons, rather than merely their performance, should be our goal.[159]

Overall, we hope to have shown that we need a different science of autism than we have now. Most of all, we hope to have shown that we need detailed longitudinal, ecologically valid case studies of autistic persons that include autistic persons as co-investigators whenever possible. By this we mean not only the acceptance of first-person perceptions as valid scientific evidence, but also their active participation in the science of autism. Only after we have a sufficient number of detailed case studies of autistic persons and their lives, could we look for the meaningful similarities and differences in the observed patterns, as psychologist Howard Gardner (1997; Policastro and Gardner 1999) suggested we do in the case of exceptional individuals. This will not only enable clearing the confusion about the difference between Asperger's Disorder and Asperger syndrome, but also allow for a discovery of many more varieties of autism that may exist under the autistic umbrella.

Since many scientists, in the field of psychology in particular, do not accept case studies as "science," we cite here the Russian neuropsychologist, Alexander Luria, a great scientist who writes about classical and romantic science, two necessarily complementary orientations within science:

> Classical scholars are those who look upon events in terms of their constituent parts. Step by step they single out important units and elements until they can formulate abstract, general laws. These laws are then seen as the governing agents of the phenomena in the field under study. One outcome of this approach is the reduction of living reality with all its richness of detail to abstract schemas. The properties of the living whole are lost, which provoked Goethe to pen, "Gray is every theory, but ever green is the tree of life."
>
> Romantic scholars' traits, attitudes, and strategies are just the opposite. They do not follow the path of reductionism, which is the leading philosophy of the classical group. Romantics in science want neither to split living reality into its elementary components nor to represent the wealth of life's concrete events in abstract models that lose the properties of the phenomena themselves. It is of the utmost importance to romantics to preserve the wealth of living reality, and they aspire to a science that retains this richness. (1979, p.174)

Luria's own romantic science (Luria 1968, 1972; see also James 1902), like our study of Teodor, involved detailed longitudinal studies of unusual persons that included his own observations, autobiographical pieces, and quantitative—objective measures. Like Luria, we also believe that understanding unusual persons requires taking into account different perspectives, including their own perspective and that of those who are close to them and know them well. As Alexander Luria says, science's

> main goal is to view an event from as many perspectives as possible. The eye of science does not probe "a thing," an event isolated from other things or events. Its real object is to see and understand the way a thing or event relates to other things or events. (1979, pp.177–178)

In our study, we have considered many perspectives on Teodor and his autistic condition, and we have learned important things from all of them. This suggests that one approach is not enough to really understand a person, no matter how "good" the approach is. There are inherent limitations in any single approach and that must triangulate information from different perspectives to really understand a person—be it autistic or not.

For Teodor, his family, and school, it does not really matter whether Teodor is autistic or Asperger's; it does not even matter whether Teodor is or is not autistic. To them, Teodor is a person deserving of the same kind of care and respect that he would receive if he did not have any of these labels. Nor does it really matter to the community or society at large, to the extent that people like Teodor can contribute to our collective well-being, and that we engage them in ways that are interhuman. For example, even if her co-workers perhaps find her unusual, it has not stopped Temple Grandin from being a successful business person—and this is all that her co-workers might require of her. Nor has her autism stopped her from being a respected university professor, writer and autism advocate.

We hope nothing will stop Teodor from reaching his full potential. Let's hope the care of all those around him will allow and foster the expression of his potential in a fulfilling and productive life. Let us also hope that in the near future, science will bring more certainty about what, when, and how we could better care for Teodor and others like him.

7

Epilogue

Transfer Boy No More

Most of this book is a reworking of Ljiljana's master's thesis, written when Teodor was twelve years old. And while we worked on improving the thesis manuscript for publication over the last two years, Teodor was also working on his own "improvement." He started having a new interest—photography. First he began taking photographs of buses, trains, and planes, and slowly of other subjects such as people, animals, and buildings. He also started to be interested in web design and has since learned how to create web pages. He already has a web page of his own, on which he posts photographs of means of transportation, friends and family members, as well as photos from his family trips.

Teodor is still interested in public transit, but not with the same zeal as he was for the eight years before; it is now only one of his interests—and not even the main one, which has become photography. But none of his current interests has the intensity and quality that could be characterized as obsessive—they are truly hobbies. Most interestingly, Teodor stopped collecting transfers from the TTC and other local transits—but still keeps the transfers and tickets from new places he visits. Teodor still loves to have fun with sounds, but has complete control over when it is or is not a good time and place to engage in that kind of fun. Kevin is still Teodor's best friend, and although he does not have any new friends, he has started to invite his friends to play with him much more often and converse much more with other children. Teodor's parents continue to help fostering these interactions.

Teodor is now a high-school student and is doing very well without extra help in the classroom. However, his parents still devote a lot of their time to help Teodor achieve better in school than he would on his own. At his middle school graduation Teodor received two awards: the "Yes I Can," and the "Diamond Award" for working hard. His school marks were "around" 75 per cent.

After Ljiljana completed her study of Teodor, as part of her debriefing she explained to Teodor why she chose to write about him and what she meant by "unusualness" in her thesis title: *Perspectives on unusualness: Transfer Boy.* But before she did this, she asked Teodor whether he has ever heard the words "autism" or "Asperger syndrome." His answer was no. Ljiljana then showed him a book written for Asperger syndrome children and they read together about other children like him. During the discussion about the book, and about autism, Teodor said that he wanted to learn how to interact with other children and be "un-autistic."

Recently (February 28, 2004), when asked about whether he thinks that he has changed since he was twelve, Teodor said:

> After I learned that I am autistic, I got interested in what makes me autistic so I can improve. Before, I used to say to children, "None of your business," when they wanted to have conversation. Now, I became nice to children—wanting to have conversations and playing with them. I want to improve more in "creating a conversation" because most of the time, children start the conversation.

When we asked Teodor's best friend Kevin whether he had noticed any change in Teodor in the past few years, he said: "Oh yeah, he matured a lot, he improved a lot, he behaves more like a teenager." When asked to give some examples of this improvement, he said, "He is not collecting transfers any more – he is collecting them but is not constantly asking for them. He is not making silly noises on the buses, or in my ear. He is not constantly talking about buses. He is not bossy."

Leo Kanner believed that "type of reactions [of autistic children] to the growing awareness of their peculiarities" (1973, p.208) in the early to middle teens might be the decisive factor in determining the successful life outcome. He noticed that children who made the biggest progress were those who made a "conscious effort to do something" about their "lack of inherent sociability" (p.210). He noticed that these same children, once they "knew" that they were expected to have friends, and once they realized "their inability to form a genuine buddy-buddy relationship" (p.210), started using their preoccupations to open a door for contact. Teodor seems to be doing exactly that; Teodor's most recent autobiography (March 28, 2004), written specifically for this book,[160] testifies to that. But, most importantly, it testifies of the importance of "genuine care"—his parents' and his best friend's.

Who I Am

I am a 15-year-old grade 9 student. My hobbies are: photography, transportation, and website design. I also like to travel and visit other cities and countries.

Until I was 12 years old, I used to love going on buses, and I was going on a lot of bus trips. Right now, since the age of 13, I understood that going on buses just for fun is a waste of time and money, so I stopped going on buses, except when I need to go to other places through the city.

I like taking pictures of my friends, buildings and skyscrapers in cities I visit and of means of transportation. When I go on vacations, I take a lot of pictures of buildings in the cities I visit.

I have my own website. I put pictures of means of transportation in one section, and in another section, pictures from my trips, other cities, and of my friends – If they don't mind. If you want to visit my website, the address is… I've recently learned how to take better pictures.

I also like playing with my friends. I invite my friends to my house,[161] we play cards and I have a train that my friends like to play with a lot. Right now, the train is in the basement of my house, on a large table. The train is operating on tracks. The tracks have a loop around the table. Me, my friend and my father are building a mountain "in the loop". It is still under construction. My friends also like when we take pictures and I put some of those pictures on the website. Sometimes, we go together skating, swimming and to the movies or to have lunch.

When I wasn't behaving like I should behave, until I was 12 years old, my best friend, Kevin, used to help me by telling me to stop or listen to the adult. He understands me.

In school, my favorite class is Geography. My marks so far are "around" 80%.

Appendix A

Method of this Study

In this book we used a method typical of many case studies. A case study is an empirical method of inquiry that investigates a phenomenon of interest in its real-life context by coordinating multiple sources of evidence (Yin 1989). In psychology, case studies have been particularly recommended by Gordon Allport (1961) and Howard Gardner (2002) as a way of studying persons and their unique ways of being. Allport (1961) called this method the *idiographic approach* and recommended using interviews, observation, and the analysis of letters or diaries as its principal sources of information. He contrasted this method with that of studying groups (i.e., the *nomothetic approach*) which uses group experimental research design in the search for general "laws" of mind and behavior.

There are different types of case studies. The most common distinction made is between *quantitative* and *qualitative* studies (Bogdan and Biklen 1998; Stake 1995, 2000; Yin 1989). Quantitative case studies are studies in which specific measurements of the case are used as sources of evidence (Yin 1989) to clarify the relationship between small numbers of variables (Stake 1995). The main goal of a qualitative case study is a deeper understanding and description of a particular case with the emphasis on its wholeness (Stake 1995). Qualitative case studies draw from a variety of research methods: phenomenological, ethnographic, biographic, naturalistic, and holistic.

Although some believe that any particular case is not necessarily representative of a population of individuals, we feel that this objection misses the point. Life is lived in the particular; we are not instances of some group. This is why Gardner (2002), for example, says that we need to develop detailed cases of particular individuals, and only when we have many of them will it be interesting to consider if there are characteristics that remain true of them as a group. We believe that while it is sometimes problematic to generalize from one individual to the characteristics of a group, it is equally problematic to generalize from the prototypical characteristics of a group to specifics of any particular individual. Certainly, at a minimum, both kinds of studies mutually inform each other.

Most of the data for this study were collected during a four-month period (from May to August 2001) in the context of regular visits of Ljiljana with Teodor and his family. The main sources of information were interviews, psychological tests and questionnaires, participant observations, documents (formal and informal), and artifacts made by Teodor.

At the time that data were collected for this project, the first author, Ljiljana, had known Teodor and his parents for five years and had worked with Teodor in different settings. She had been his after-school program instructor, summer program inclusion facilitator, social skills group leader, therapist and tutor. She was then (and still is) working with him as a tutor and therapist. Then, she met with him twice a week for two to three hours, and now they meet once a week for three hours—either at his or her home. Ljiljana has known Teodor's best friend for three years and he has been involved in a number of planned activities with Teodor (such as visits to educational and fun places, homework, and various activities just for fun and conversation). Ljiljana has also met Teodor's teaching assistant on a few occasions. The second author, Michel, was the supervisor for Ljiljana's master's thesis, which served as the basis for this book.

Interviews with Teodor were of two kinds: informal and formal. Informal interviews were in a form of casual conversation; formal interviews involved two structured questionnaires, the Self-Understanding Interview (Damon and Hart 1988) and clinical interview based on the Self-Perception Profile for Children (Harter 1985). Some of these interviews were conducted at Teodor's and some at Ljiljana's home. Interviews with other participants (Teodor's family members and the teaching assistant) were all semistructured. Interviews with Teodor's family members were conducted in Teodor's home in a relaxed and informal conversational atmosphere. Family members did not hear other members' interviews, except for Teodor's mother, who interpreted/translated the interviews with Teodor's grandparents (since they do not speak English). Teodor's mother was interviewed before the interviews with Teodor's grandparents took place. The interviews with Teodor's grandparents were approximately 15 minutes long, and with his parents 50 minutes. The main focus of the questions asked was on family members' experiences and perceptions about Teodor's way of being. The semi-structured interview with Teodor's teaching assistant took approximately 25 minutes and was conducted in Teodor's school. The purpose of this interview was to collect data about Teodor's way of being in a social and educational environment. Interviews with all participants were audio-recorded and transcribed.

Two psychometric tests were used in this study: the Wechsler Intelligence Scale for Children—Third Edition (WISC-III), administered to Teodor, and the Self-Perception Profile for Children (Harter 1985), administered to Teodor, his parents, and the teaching assistant. In addition, observations of Teodor were made in real-life everyday settings. Also, four types of documents and artifacts were used in the study: Teodor's letters, postcards and e-mails to Liljana, his several autobiographical and biographical essays, as well as his other writings and drawings; his written school assignments; photographs of artifacts made by him, such as toys and paper models of bus stations; his official school and medical records, from which the data on school achievements and the psychiatric diagnosis, neurological and neurophysiological functioning, and the data from functional and structural brain imaging were taken. In addition, Teodor's best friend's autobiographical and biographical essays were also obtained for comparison purposes.

The case study we presented here thus represents a combination of qualitative (intrinsic and instrumental) and quantitative case studies.

Case studies have often been criticized by saying that the researcher's subjectivity necessarily biases data collection and interpretation (Bogdan and Biklen 1998; Kvale 1996; Stake 1995, 2000). However, qualitative researchers not only take into account their subjectivity and acknowledge it; they also have specific procedures of dealing with it through "triangulation" (Stake 1995, 2000).

Two of the most recognized triangulation procedures are "data source triangulation" (which refers to data collection in different times, spaces and contexts) and "methodological triangulation" (which refers to data collection using multiple methods such as observation, interview and document review). There is also a procedure for triangulating the obtained data and its interpretation. This procedure is called "member checking" and involves having participants examine rough drafts of those parts of the report that concern their actions and words. The subjects are asked to review the report for accuracy and make suggestions for improvement in interpretation. Finally, the case study report must include sufficient detail so that others can draw their own conclusions, which may not be the same as the researcher's (Stake 1995, 2000).

In an effort to achieve interpretative validity in the study, we employed qualitative triangulation (Stake 1995, 2000). The following data checks were employed: (1) multiple data-gathering techniques (interviews, observation, and document and record analysis); (2) multiple data sources; and (3) discussions with everyone involved about our interpretations throughout the book.

Of course, our story about Teodor is only one possible story about him. Ljiljana chose to collect data on what interested her, and what she believes is most important about Teodor's way of being. Therefore, this project is, in a sense, a documentary of both the person observed and the observer. Another researcher studying the same case might obtain different findings or emphasize different aspects of them in his or her interpretation.

Qualitative researchers argue that in a real-life context it is neither possible nor necessary to obtain data that admits of only a single interpretation (as long as the data and interpretations obtained by different researchers are not contradictory or incompatible), since there are myriad aspects of any given case that could be of interest to different researchers (Bogdan and Biklen 1998). Someone else could certainly collect different data about Teodor and tell a different story—but not, we believe, a contradictory one. Some have even argued that one of the aims of qualitative case researchers is to preserve the "multiple realities" that are characteristic of human life (Stake 1995, p.12).

Appendix B

Diagnostic Criteria for Autistic Disorder

A. A total of six (or more) items from (1), (2), and (3), with at least two from (1), and one each from (2) and (3):

(1) qualitative impairment in social interaction, as manifested by at least two of the following:

(a) marked impairment in the use of multiple nonverbal behaviors such as eye-to-eye gaze, facial expression, body postures, and gestures to regulate social interaction

(b) failure to develop peer relationships appropriate to developmental level

(c) a lack of spontaneous seeking to share enjoyment, interests, or achievements with other people (e.g., by a lack of showing, bringing, or pointing out objects of interest)

(d) lack of social or emotional reciprocity

(2) qualitative impairments in communication as manifested by at least one of the following:

(a) delay in, or total lack of, the development of spoken language (not accompanied by an attempt to compensate through alternative modes of communication such as gesture or mime)

(b) in individuals with adequate speech, marked impairment in the ability to initiate or sustain a conversation with others

(c) stereotyped and repetitive use of language or idiosyncratic language

(d) lack of varied, spontaneous make-believe play or social imitative play appropriate to developmental level

(3) restricted repetitive and stereotyped patterns of behavior, interests, and activities, as manifested by at least one of the following:

(a) encompassing preoccupation with one or more stereotyped and restricted patterns of interest that is abnormal either in intensity or focus

(b) apparently inflexible adherence to specific, nonfunctional routines or rituals

(c) stereotyped and repetitive motor mannerisms (e.g., hand or finger flapping or twisting, or complex whole-body movements)

(d) persistent preoccupation with parts of objects

B. Delays or abnormal functioning in at least one of the following areas, with onset prior to age 3 years: (1) social interaction, (2) language as used in social communication, or (3) symbolic or imaginative play.

C. The disturbance is not better accounted for by Rett's Disorder or Childhood Disintegrative Disorder.

Reproduced with permission from the *Diagnostic and Statistical Manual of Mental Disorders*, Text Revision, Copyright 2000. American Psychiatric Association (APA 2000, p.75).

Appendix C

Diagnostic Criteria for Asperger's Disorder

A. Qualitative impairment in social interaction, as manifested by at least two of the following:

  (1) marked impairment in the use of multiple nonverbal behaviors such as eye-to-eye gaze, facial expression, body postures, and gestures to regulate social interaction
  (2) failure to develop peer relationships appropriate to developmental level
  (3) a lack of spontaneous seeking to share enjoyment, interests, or achievements with other people (e.g., by a lack of showing, bringing, or pointing out objects of interest to other people)
  (4) lack of social or emotional reciprocity

B. Restricted repetitive and stereotyped patterns of behavior, interests, and activities, as manifested by at least one of the following:

  (1) encompassing preoccupation with one or more stereotyped and restricted patterns of interest that is abnormal either in intensity or focus
  (2) apparently inflexible adherence to specific, nonfunctional routines or rituals
  (3) stereotyped and repetitive motor mannerisms (e.g., hand or finger flapping or twisting, or complex whole-body movements)
  (4) persistent preoccupation with parts of objects

C. The disturbance causes clinically significant impairment in social, occupational, or other important areas of functioning.

D. There is no clinically significant general delay in language (e.g., single words used by age 2 years, communicative phrases used by 3 years).

E. There is no clinically significant delay in cognitive development or in the development of age-appropriate self-help skills, adaptive behavior (other than in social interaction), and curiosity about the environment in childhood.

F. Criteria are not met for another specific Pervasive Developmental Disorder or Schizophrenia.

Reproduced with permission from the *Diagnostic and Statistical Manual of Mental Disorders*, Text Revision, Copyright 2000. American Psychiatric Association (APA 2000, p.84).

Notes

1 Swiss psychiatrist Eugen Bleuler coined the term autism, from the Greek word "autos" for "self", to refer to unrealistic thinking and the loss of contact with reality in schizophrenia (1916/1951).

2 Capital letters are used throughout to denote formal diagnostic labels.

3 She means that life in Romania would be quieter for her without Teodor.

4 TTC (The Toronto Transit Commission) refers to the Toronto public transportation system that includes buses, street-cars, trains and subways.

5 Refers to their recent vacation in Mexico, and her attempt to point out and explain to Teodor what poverty is, and realizing that he had absolutely no interest in the subject.

6 Since interviews with Teodor's grandparents were much shorter than those with Teodor's parents, many issues (e.g., those involving school) did not come up.

7 The omitted parts pertain to the detailed description of Teodor's performance with regard to specific topics studied.

8 It may be important to note that Teodor had another teacher for this subject.

9 Note that none of the areas was assessed to be at the lowest level, i.e., as "needs improvement."

10 Note that this was the semester to which Teodor's mother referred as "experimental," that is, in which she tried to "minimize" her involvement with Teodor's homework, and which, according to her, had some negative effects on Teodor's school marks.

11 Another case is that of an autistic person with an intense and prolonged interest in watches and time who as an adult developed a computer program that can calculate the seconds that passed at any given time since the millennium began (Burack 2002).

12 This is not unusual; seizure and autism frequently co-occur, with estimates of prevalence ranging from 5 per cent to 38.3 per cent (see Tuchman and Rapin 2002 for a recent review).

13 This condition was first described sixty years ago by the American psychiatrist Leo Kanner (1943), who noticed that a group of children he treated at the time all shared the same set of characteristics: impaired social interaction and communication, repetitive behavior, a rigid need for routine and impaired language. He termed this condition *early infantile autism.*

14 Asperger's Disorder was thought to be first described by Austrian pediatrician Hans Asperger (1944/1991) at almost exactly the same time as Leo Kanner described early infantile autism. Asperger and Kanner described children who exhibited a similar pattern of behaviors and both independently referred to these children encountered in their clinical practice as autistic. More precisely, Asperger referred to a condition he described as *autistic psychopathy.* Both Kanner and Asperger referred to the Swiss psychiatrist Eugen Bleuler. However, unlike Kanner's children, Asperger's children (all boys) started showing problems at a later age and usually their speech was not delayed, although they had greater motor difficulties. Asperger wrote in German and was largely unknown to the English-speaking world before Lorna Wing's paper (1981). In 1990 *Asperger's syndrome* was included in the official taxonomy of the ICD-10 (*International Classification of Diseases,* WHO 1990). Four years later, this condition was also recognized by the American Psychiatric Association and was included in the official psychiatric classification system under the name of Asperger's Disorder (APA 1994). Ironically, Sula Wolff (1995) has recently discovered that a Russian neurologist, Ewa Ssucharewa, described a group of children with very similar characteristics in 1926.

15 Christopher Gillberg use his own criteria which instead of language delay require "speech and language peculiarities" and are actually closer to Asperger's original descriptions.

16 Although having a diagnosis of a "handicap condition" was somewhat beneficial to Teodor and his family, the benefits did not meet his parents' expectations. Initially, the diagnosis provided an interpretation of their son's unusual behavior, but it also gave them a short-lived hope that it would lead to the

prescription of an appropriate treatment as is often the case with other medical conditions. However, there is no therapy that can make their son "autism free." Interventions, if chosen properly, might make Teodor appear less autistic and function better in the society. But, choosing the right intervention is not an easy task. First, these interventions are numerous and *scientific* evidence for their effectiveness is scarce (for recent reviews on the available treatment options see Howlin 1998, and Trevarthen *et al.* 1998; and on treatment guidelines, Klin and Volkmar 2000). Second, not all interventions are equally suited for all subgroups of children within the autistic spectrum, nor to all children within the same subgroup. This means that not all children with Asperger's Disorder would benefit equally from the same treatment. And we have seen from the example of treatments prescribed to Teodor, behavioral management and social skills training, that they were not particularly well suited to Teodor and his difficulties. The behavioral management intervention program that Teodor and his mother attended, also on advice from the psychiatrist, was designed for children with behavior disorders—not for autistic children. And even though it provided Teodor's mother with some useful strategies, the "teaching strategy" was not particularly well suited to Teodor's learning needs; there was no provision of visual (Hodgdon 1995; Klin andVolkmar 2000) or any other learning support (Quill 1995). The missing element here was not the lack of services, but rather the lack of a more comprehensive assessment of Teodor's specific needs. As Lorna Wing noted, the "DSM-IV subgroups are of no use" for planning intervention of designing services (2000, p.428). She argued for the value of more descriptive classification along three dimensions: quality of social interaction, verbal communication, and nonverbal and practical skills, which could serve as the starting point for choosing the most appropriate intervention. Third, intervention for autism/Asperger's Disorder should be a treatment package that includes a combination of treatments for different areas of functioning: social, communication and language, behavior, sensory and motor.

17 None of the reviewed studies focused specifically on children with Asperger syndrome, although many children with Asperger syndrome were included in them.

18 Examples of adult-mediated direct teaching of understanding the mental states of others (Howlin, Baron-Cohen, and Hadwin 1999); or Carol Gray's "Social Stories" (1993, 1994, 1998) which involve the use of individualized stories that, in addition to the instructions for specific situations (such as recess, party or a group activity), have a description of the situation and the reactions and feelings of others who are involved. Readers interested in social skills interventions for autistic children are referred to recent reviews by Tony Attwood (2000), Rhea Paul (2003) and Sally Rogers (2000).

19 While some studies found movement difficulties to be significantly more present in Asperger syndrome than in autism (e.g., Gillberg 1989; Green *et al.* 2002; Klin *et al.* 1995), others did not (Ghaziuddin *et al.* 1994; Manjiviona and Prior 1995).

20 When we consider the previously discussed and other conceptual and methodological limitations of studies investigating Asperger syndrome, it should not be surprising that the results are contradictory (see Smith 2000).

21 In this book, the term Asperger's Disorder is used only to refer to Teodor's formal psychiatric diagnosis and the discussion of it in this chapter.

22 Canadian norms.

23 The test was administered in the Counseling and Psychoeducational Clinic at the Ontario Institute for Studies in Education at the University of Toronto.

24 According to the instructions of the test administration, the examiner is not allowed to change the wordings of the instructions, but can emphasize by intonation.

25 Interestingly, some researchers have suggested that the opposite is the case (Szatmari 2000).

26 The interview with Teodor's mother was conducted before the intelligence testing.

27 Children were 6; 6 to 20; 9 years old. All participants functioned intellectually above the retarded range—full scale IQ70. The groups were matched on chronological age, gender, and intellectual ability.

28 The first psychological experimental studies on autism were conducted twenty years after Kanner's identification of the autistic condition (Hermelin and O'Connor 1964, 1970).

29 Thus, in some contexts, global processing of autistic persons was impaired (see Plaisted, Swettenham and Rees 1999 [the divided attention task; experiment 2]; Rinehart *et al.* 2000), while in others it was intact (e.g., Mottron *et al.* 1999; Ozonoff *et al.* 1994; Plaisted *et al.* 1999 [the selective attention task; experiment 1]).

30 Some experts consider some aspects of attention and memory to be executive functions; most would agree that attention and memory overlap with executive functions (Pennington and Ozonoff 1996).

31 This is usually measured by a neuropsychological test of conceptual problem solving called the Wisconsin Card Sorting Test, in which subjects are required to sort a set of cards by a rule that they must deduce from the feedback provided by the examiner. When the sorting rule changes, some autistic persons find it difficult to abandon the previously correct strategy of sorting cards by one particular feature (e.g., colour) and begin sorting them by another (e.g., shape). The planning aspect of executive function is typically assessed by the Tower of Hanoi or the Tower of London tasks in which subjects have to move discs from one peg to the other (using three pegs) according to a specific set of rules and with the goal of producing a specific sequence. The *inhibition* aspect of executive function is commonly assessed using the Stroop task, in which the subjects are first asked to read a list of colour names printed in coloured ink (e.g., the word "red" printed in red ink) and then to name the colour ink in which the words are printed (e.g., to say "red" for the word "blue" printed in red ink). However, there are many other tasks that are used in assessing executive function, each tapping a somewhat different aspect of it.

32 In spite of Kanner's (1943) initial view that autism is a disorder of an innate inability to form an "affective contact with people" (p.250), the first experimental studies to investigate social and emotional aspects of autism were conducted some forty years later—during the first wave of cognitive studies as part of the "cognitive revolution".

33 Another popular false belief task is the Ice-Cream Van Task (Baron-Cohen 1989a), a more advanced, second-order false-belief task—typically solved by children of 6–8 years (Bowler 1992). In this task, too, the story is enacted with two dolls, Mary and John. Mary and John are in the park when the ice-cream van comes and they both see it. Then Mary goes home to get some money, and John sees the ice-cream van move to the church. Mary unexpectedly sees the ice-cream van at the church too. John looks for Mary and is told that she has gone for an ice cream. The child is then asked where John thinks Mary went. Experimental studies that used this task found that some autistic children pass this "second-order ToM task"—usually those with Asperger syndrome (Bowler 1992; Ozonoff, Rogers, and Pennington 1991).

34 There have also been a few studies that used Piagetian tasks such as object permanence (Adrien, Martineau, and Barthelemy 1995) or perspective taking (Dawson and Fernald 1987), and sensorimotor tasks (Morgan *et al.* 1989) as well as many other tasks that psychologists use to test cognition in different knowledge domains such as biology, physics, and mathematics (see, for example, Peterson and Siegal 1997).

35 Depending on their theoretical framework, different experts stress different aspects of this capacity. For example, Simon Baron-Cohen emphasizes the cognitive aspect of joint attention and considers it a precursor to understanding others' minds and solving standard theory of mind tasks (Baron-Cohen 1995) while others stress its emotional (e.g., Mundy 1995) and attentional aspect.

36 This instrument is a forced-choice questionnaire with 36 items grouped into six subscales that yields separate measures of one's perceptions of competence in each of six domains. The child is posed problems such as "Some kids have a lot of friends, BUT other kids don't have very many friends." The child first decides which of these children are most like her or him, and then decides whether the chosen description is "sort of true" or "really true" for her or him. Each answer is scored from 1 to 4—four indicates "the most adequate self-judgment" and one—"the least adequate self-judgment" (Harter 1985, p.12). Harter found that the mean score of typically developing children is around 3, or more specifically, for grade six boys, the mean scores range from 2.85—on behavioral conduct subscale—to 3.08—on athletic competence subscale.

37 This questionnaire has 15 questions, three from each of the five specific domains. Susan Harter (1985), who designed this instrument, does not believe that global self-worth can be evaluated by others and so they are not asked questions about the child's global self-worth. Adult evaluators are instead asked questions about the child's "actual behavior" such as "This child has a lot of friends, or this child doesn't have many friends." After deciding which of these statements applies to the child, they also decide whether the chosen description is "sort of true" or "really true" of the child. The answers are scored the same way as children's answers—from 1 to 4.

38 Though this instrument is called the Teacher's Rating Scale for Children's Actual Behavior, suggesting that it is meant to be used by teachers, instructions in the instrument manual allow it to be administered to any individual who knows the child (Harter 1985, p.12).

39 This is the only domain where there was an absolute agreement among the three adult raters.

40 However, according to adults who know him, he is very adequate (score of 4) in one domain (physical appearance), somewhat competent/adequate in two (scholastic competence, behavioral conduct) and somewhat inadequate/incompetent in two (social acceptance and athletic competence). And we have also seen that in most (i.e., four, or all but one) of the domains Teodor's and others' ratings fell into opposing categories. Only their ratings of Teodor's physical appearance fell into the same general category (i.e., adequate) but still differed in the subcategory into which they fell (i.e., "somewhat" or "very").

41 In her instruction manual for the Self-Perception Profile for Children, Harter (1985) recommends conducting such an interview with atypical children.

42 Question # 34.

43 Question # 10—score of 4.

44 Questions # 16 and 22—score of 1.

45 Teodor's answers to questions # 4, 16, and 34 were probed on three different days.

46 Question # 16.

47 It should be noted that Teodor does have a somewhat rough skin.

48 Question # 9—score of 1.

49 Question # 3—score of 2.

50 Question # 15—score of 4.

51 Question # 8—score of 3.

52 However, on another occasion, his answer on the same question was "five or more." He also named six children that he considers his friends, and provided the explanations as to why they are his friends.

53 Question # 14—score of 1. We also see that his scores vary (1–3), even when evaluating the same aspect of social acceptance—namely the number of friends he has and he would like to have.

54 Question # 14.

55 By "looking at pictures" Teodor means that sometime during the schoolwork, the TTC pictures come to his mind and interfere with his work.

56 This statement is similar to the one by Teodor's grandfather who said that children at Teodor's age have other interests than TTC.

57 One of Teodor's poems about himself appears in the next chapter.

58 Question # 11.

59 Teodor said he knows that he is annoying, for example, to Kevin, when he tells him "Next trip cancelled!" or "None of your business!" Or to other children when he was picking his nose ("before").

60 Question # 35—score of 2.

61 Question # 12.

62 On another occasion he compared the speed with which the girl that sat next to him on the test answered the test questions and said that he wished he could answer the questions that fast.

63 We used the new (1985) version, which has two new subscales: physical appearance and behavioral conduct. In addition, physical competence is now renamed athletic competence (with some new questions added).

64 However, there is an exception, namely, if girls would come and ask him to play. "I won't say, 'No, later'—I won't say that *with* them."

65 Another example of playing according to a time schedule could be found in his brief description of skating when he "was a train," and had to stay at the "station" for the required time period, "approximately six minutes."

66 It is interesting to compare Teodor's reaction to his friend's reaction when he interrupted him in what he was doing. He said, "I was gonna ask him [...]I just said, 'Victor,' when he was *just looking at how people are playing,* and he said, 'Can't you see I'm busy?' That's not the reason to be busy." Even more interesting is his expectation of the way the teacher could help him. He added: "and I had to tell the teacher, and the teacher—and I was hoping to say, 'Excuse me, why do you say that?'—I was hoping that the teacher would say that, 'Answer his question now'—when I told on him I was hoping that the teacher says that."

67 He said he learned this distinction from the teacher.

68 The reason for fighting in the bus is "to catch the first seat."

69 Teodor also talked about other things children do (to him) that he does not like. For example, he said, "One time I left a pen somewhere when I was climbing up, and someone took it, and he ran away with it" or "Sometimes people, like, crowd around me...and they say, 'Hey what are you doing?' when I'm trying to draw something."

70 Note that there are specific rules that his friends have to follow on these trips. For example, "No talking when the train is moving" since Teodor likes to listen to the sounds that the moving train makes.

71 In a study by Chandler *et al.*, typically developing children were engaged in a play situation involving deception, rather than in verbal deception tasks.

72 This instrument is a semi-structured interview designed to tap children and adolescents' understanding of themselves. It has seven core items (i.e., self-definition, self-evaluation, self in past and future, self-interests, continuity, agency, and distinctness), each consisting of a question or a set of questions and adequate probes. The first four items focus on what is in psychological literature known as self-as-object, and the last three on self-as-subject. Children are asked questions such as: What kind of person are you? What else are you? Why is it important that you're—? The unit of scoring is a chunk, which is defined as "*one self-characteristic* mentioned by the subject during the interview; and all the subject's statements, whether spontaneous or in response to the interviewer's probe questions, that explicate the meaning or importance of that characteristic" (Damon and Hart 1988, p.83). After all responses are chunked, they are categorized according to the aspects of self that children mentioned, i.e., physical, active, psychological or social self. Finally, children's self-statements are assigned to the appropriate developmental level (for details, see Damon and Hart 1988).

73 According to Damon and Hart, self-statements in which children refer to mental processes are psychological self-scheme.

74 When during this interview children describe themselves in terms of their associations with family, friends or other persons, or by their membership, their responses are scored as social self-scheme.

75 Eighteen, thirteen and five times, respectively.

76 It is important to note a difference between "sociability" and social participation as fulfilling an institutional role (e.g., being an engineer or a bus driver) in which one acts because one has certain knowledge or credentials. Even in self-statements in which Teodor mentions different social activities he expects to do in the future when he becomes an engineer, a bus driver, or a caretaker, he does not define himself in terms of these activities, but rather by his membership of the group of engineers, bus drivers or caretakers.

77 Responses in which children refer to their activities, performed or expected ones, are scored as "active self-scheme."

78 Responses in which children refer to their physical attributes such as one's size, gender, race, distinctive bodily features and age, or their possessions are scored as "physical self-scheme."

79 The level for this response could not be determined because Teodor was not specifically probed about it.

80 The levels are: (1) *categorical*—on which children can identify the group of children to which they belong such as boy, five-year-old, big, etc.—but are not able to draw any personal meaning of this membership; (2) *comparative assessment*, which emerges during mid-childhood and is characterized by children's comparisons of themselves with other people; (3) *interpersonal implications*—which emerges in later childhood and early adolescence and is recognized by children's reference to the manner of their interaction with others; and (4) *systematic beliefs and plans*, which emerges in late adolescence and is characterized by a systematic conception of oneself based on "philosophical or moral belief systems, ideological choices, or any variety of personal goals" (Damon and Hart 1988, p.67).

81 The TTC refers to public transit in Toronto, while Go Transit refers to public transit in nearby cities.

82 Nine and five responses, respectively.

83 The mean mental age of the autistic participants was obtained from performance on the British Picture Vocabulary Test. Although we cannot compare Teodor directly on this measure, his WISC-III score seems to place him at about the high-end of the range of these children.

84 It is important to note that the range of such statements made by individual subjects in Lee and Hobson's study was 0–6, while the range for autistic children was 0–3.

85 Twenty questions (without probes) about self-as-object and self-as-subject were asked during this interview.

86 Teodor used the word *know* (and its derivatives) the most often—54 times during 30 minutes of this interview (excluding the "I don't know" replies). In addition to being very knowledgeable in—or in his terms "smart about"—public transit, he also thinks that he is smart about other things, such as math—percents and additions in particular. In his judgment, he "may be *smart* about both equally, like half about that and half about that, or maybe 75 per cent about buses and 25 per cent about *knowing* things." In general, *learning* and *studying* (about both public transit and "other things") seem to be important activities to Teodor. He used words learning and studying often too (17 times) and the word *taught* once (to refer to what he learned about transfers from his mother).

87 This is based on evidence that the rate of autism is much higher in autistic identical than in non-identical twins. It has been estimated that in a family with one autistic child, the chances of having a second child with autism are 50 to 100 times greater (i.e., 1 in 20) than in the general population (i.e., 1 in 1000; Bailey *et al.* 1995).

88 It has been estimated that in 10 per cent of cases autism is associated with other known neurological disorders, such as fragile X syndrome, tuberous sclerosis, and phenylketonuria (Rutter *et al.* 1994). This association of autism with different neurological disorders indicates its genetic heterogeneity (Lamb *et al.* 2000).

89 The genes investigated include RELN and HOXA1—genes involved in brain development, WNT2—a gene involved in embryogenesis, FOXP2—a gene involved in language development, 5–HTT and 5–HTR 7—two genes involved in the metabolism of the major excitatory neurotransmitter serotonin, DB—a gene involved in conversion of dopamine to norepinephrine, GABRB3—a gene for a major inhibitory neurotransmitter GABA, and GRIK2—the glutamate receptor gene, among others.

90 For a critical discussion of the findings in this area see Karmiloff-Smith (1998); for a developmental perspective on genetics and neurobiology of autism, see Koenig, Tsatsanis, and Volkmar (2001).

91 A drug used to treat epilepsy.

92 A drug used by pregnant women to alleviate morning sickness.

93 Major sources of mercury, for children, are the preservative Thimerosal (which, until recently, was added to many vaccines), contaminated foods (such as fish), skin creams, and infant teething powders (Bernard *et al.* 2001).

94 Here again, Nelson Goodman's "one finds what one looks for" might shed some light on these results.

95 Interestingly, even when different studies find the same brain structure to be atypical, findings about the nature of this atypicality vary across studies. For example, some studies investigating the amygdala volume in autistic individuals found that it is decreased (Aylward *et al.* 1999), increased (Howard *et al.* 2000), or not different from control subjects (Haznedar *et al.* 2000).

96 Structural MRI uses magnets to reveal slices of the brain (for more details see Uttal 2001).

97 This kind of study involves cytological analysis of autopsy brain tissue. So far, only about 30 autistic brains have been examined (Lord *et al.* 2000).

98 This brain structure was previously thought to be involved only in coordinating movements, but was recently found to modulate many cognitive processes, such as attention, memory and complex problem solving (for more details see Allen *et al.* 1997).

99 In short, these techniques measure changes in blood flow through areas of the brain or brain metabolism (e.g., glucose utilization), and have been used as indirect measure of brain activity. However, while fMRI is noninvasive, PET and SPECT involve radiation and (often) sedation. For more details about functional neuroimaging and other brain measurement techniques see recent reviews by Marcus Raichle (2001) and William Uttal (2001).

100 However, there is a controversy over the exact function of the fusiform gyrus. Some researchers have argued that it plays a general role in processing of visual information for all objects, including faces, (1) for which there was a sufficient experience to allow processing to become automated, and (2) when one is interested in the unique identity of objects. Therefore, according to these researchers, it is better described as an "expert area" (Gauthier and Tarr 1997; Tarr and Cheng 2003; Tarr and Gauthier 2000).

101 ERP waves consist of a number of different components each of which reflects different sensory and cognitive processes. For details, see Uttal (2001).

102 Some studies also investigated the association between autism and a number of serotonin related genes (Veenstra-Vanderweele and Cook 2003); however, the findings are inconclusive (e.g., Betancur *et al.* 2002).

103 Cerebrospinal fluid circulates through and around the brain and the spinal cord.

104 Elevated blood serotonin levels are not specific to autism; they are also found in schizophrenia, and severe mental retardation (Hanley, Stahl, and Freedman 1977; Stahl *et al.* 1983).

105 There are several reasons why measures of levels of blood serotonin may not be good indicators of its concentrations in the brain. This is because serotonin is produced both in the intestines and in the brain; however, serotonin from blood cannot pass through the filtering cells called the "blood-brain barrier" although its precursor can. Therefore, using measures of serotonin levels in the blood as an indicator of central activity has to be established as valid first; the available evidence suggests that there is no relationship between serotonin measures in the two environments (Elliott and Ciaranello 1987; Sarrias *et al.* 1990; Strawn *et al.* 2002).

106 Importantly, two out of nine children had the opposite pattern of low serotonin production.

107 Neuropeptides may act as neurotransmitters or neuromodulators.

108 Neurotrophins (also called growth factors) are substances that regulate neuronal growth, survival and connections during early brain development.

109 It is of interest that it was also noted at that time that "He also appears to have long-standing socialization difficulties." However, no further assessment had been recommended.

110 Brain tumor near the hypothalamus (the brain region involved in regulation of hormone production) which is associated with seizures and precocious (early) puberty.

111 It is difficult to compare Teodor's SPECT scans with those of other autistic children because Teodor was also diagnosed with seizure, and even though many other children with autism also have seizures (as we mentioned earlier), and are commonly included in studies that used SPECT scans, there is no study that compared SPECT scans of autistic subjects with seizures and without them. In fact, several studies included different comorbid conditions including epilepsy and mental retardation (although not all studies specified which comorbid conditions were present). Importantly, Mountz and his colleagues did not specify comorbid conditions present in autistic subjects in their study.

112 Only two studies found structural atypicalities in the basal ganglia—each in two different nuclei (Gaffney *et al.* 1989; Sears *et al.* 1999).

113 This is according to the recent review by Nathalie Boddaert and Mônica Zilbovicius (2002), and not according to the original paper by James Mountz and his colleagues (1995) in which neurological conditions of autistic subjects were not specified. We assume that the reviewers of this paper had acquired additional information from the authors.

114 What is said in this section, and all subsequent sections, refers specifically to persons diagnosed with high-functioning autism or Asperger's Disorder. However, for reasons of brevity we will continue to refer to them as autistic, as they themselves do.

115 Two items from Autism Network International's philosophy are good illustrations of Jim's own view on autism: "Supports for autistic people should be aimed at helping them to compensate, navigate, and function in the world, not at changing them into non-autistic people or isolating them from the world" and "Autistic people have characteristically autistic styles of relating to others, which should be respected and appreciated rather than modified to make them 'fit in.'"

116 Interestingly, as its subtitle indicates, this book is not merely an autobiography, but a guide for children diagnosed with Asperger syndrome, their parents, and professionals based on his experience of what it feels like to be autistic.

117 We specifically quote passages with similarities or relevance to Teodor.

118 Jack's mother said the same about Jack: "He enjoys the companionship of his own voice" (Dewey 1991, p.204).

119 In fact, many of them diagnosed themselves, by reading or watching movies or TV shows.

120 This description is very similar to that of the psychiatrist Christopher Gillberg's (1991) description of the case III: 2—the "little professor"—who at twelve years of age also discovered that he "has" Asperger syndrome. This boy found a leaflet for parents about Asperger syndrome in Gillberg's office and, as soon as he started reading it, remarked, "It seems I have AS [Asperger syndrome]!" As he read more, he exclaimed, "By golly, I do have AS. Wait till my father hears about this! ... Now I can tell my classmates the reason I pace the school-yard briskly ten times up and down each break all the year round is I have AS" (p.138).

121 It is important to clarify this point, since it might be taken as an example of teasing—and it is not. When asked whether he thinks that other children were trying to annoy him on purpose or they just like to sit

on that chair, regardless of whether he is there or not, he said, "Oh, yeah, *everybody* likes to sit on it. It stands on wheels and it rotates."

122 Sometimes information about the change is indicated on the transfer (e.g., when the place on it marked as "spc" [for "special"] is punched), but usually it is not—and even when it is, Teodor still would want to know exactly what had been changed—which is never indicated on the transfer. Interestingly, it is these special transfers that are given a prominent place among the transfers in Teodor's collection.

123 This was an appropriate question since it was Ljiljana's first day as a graduate student (which also partly explains why she did not reply right away as she usually did).

124 Note that this is the trip Teodor's father promised to Teodor if he gets good marks in school.

125 None of Teodor's writings were corrected for spelling or any other mistakes.

126 Teodor seems to recall that his teacher gave him only a limited time to write his answers.

127 When asked what he means by "normal face," he wrote, "his face is not ugly, [or] brown… Normal like Lilliana's face."

128 Both spelling and punctuation mistakes were corrected in order to allow for better readability.

129 Other ways, mentioned earlier, include taking public transit trips, copying the information in special notebooks, or reading the brochures.

130 A content analysis of Teodor's essay revealed that he used 65 per cent of all the words (or 157 out of 242 words) to describe his main interest, 19 per cent of words (or 45 words) to describe his second interest (i.e., watching the movies), and 16 per cent of words (or 40 words) to describe his "job" (9 per cent, or 22 words) and visits to Ontario Science Centre (7 per cent, or 18 words). Thus, he spent more time (and words) describing his main interest than all other areas of interest combined. Consequently, Teodor's descriptions of different interests also differ in the details he provided about them. Thus, Teodor took his time to explain what he collects, and how he plays public transit games, but did not do so for his visits to the Ontario Science Centre: for him, it was not important to explain how he plays there, and so he just mentions the activity of playing. And even though he says he "love[s]" his job, he did not go into any detail about what it is that he does, or loves about it. On the other hand, he did find it necessary to mention what it is about movies that he likes. And here, again, we find public transit (i.e., airplanes), and interesting things to repeat (i.e., to have fun with sounds). Therefore, one may take these differences as an indicator of the centrality of the interest in public transit in Teodor's life. And even though Teodor did not elaborate a lot on his having "fun with sounds," the fact that it seems to persist in spite of "punishment" also seems to indicate its importance.

131 It is important to note that Teodor is fully aware of the imaginary nature of his imaginary friends.

132 Vygotsky wrote, "What the child can do in cooperation today he can do alone tomorrow" (1934/1986, p.188).

133 In line with Freeman and Brockmeier's (2001) conception of autobiographical narratives as consisting of both spoken and written, and both cohesive and fragmentary, autobiographical material, we will treat all of Teodor's self-statements as self-narratives.

134 But we do want to emphasize that there are also many differences among these accounts.

135 Sean's mother, who co-authored the auto/biography book with her son, wrote that Sean liked to "insert…long words into every conversation: e.g., 'carbamylachloride,' 'fluorophosphate'" (Barron and Barron 2002, p.197). This could be related to Teodor's "fun with sounds" and the pleasure some sounds/sound combinations can elicit.

136 She also said, "Other children played school, mothers and fathers, doctors and nurses. Other children skipped ropes and played with balls or swap-cards. I had swap-cards. I gave them away in order to make friends, before learning that I was supposed to swap them, not give them away" (Williams 1999a, p.26).

137 Teodor said this as a spontaneous elaboration during his Damon and Hart's interview. However, when he said he wished he had more new friends, in the clinical interview, and was asked to explain why, he could not explain it. Instead, he said, "because they never played with me."

138 All these difficulties with team sports are also reported by clinicians (e.g., Attwood 1998). Tony Attwood also writes about the lack of interest in the success of one's team as another aspect of team sports that make them inaccessible for children diagnosed with Asperger syndrome.

139 Although the psychiatrist did make a note about Teodor being bullied at his previous school, when he was nine years old, this rarely, if ever, happens in Teodor's current school. It might be important to note that before Teodor moved to this school, Ljiljana went there and introduced him to his classmates,

teachers and other school staff before he came. She emphasized positive aspects of his unusualness and introduced all the behaviour that his classmates might view negatively as opposites of his positive characteristics. When at the end of this presentation Ljiljana asked his soon-to-be classmates to help him adjust to his new school, many children volunteered to help, Kevin being among them.

140 In psychiatry this is considered a thought disorder, and labeled "perseveration."

141 It should be noted that in spite of her awareness that autistic persons often acknowledge their knowledge of words having shared meanings (but still insist on using their own terms, since they convey better what they want to express or emphasize; see p.214), Happé interprets these idosyncrasies as stemming from a lack of awareness of the difference between shared and private knowledge.

142 Stands for Treatment and Education of Autistic and Related Communication Handicapped Children, an intervention approach developed in the early 1970s which emphasizes structured teaching.

143 Note that Lorna Wing (1981) proposed "lack of imagination" in autism to be one of three core impairments.

144 The list of support-groups could be found at: http://www.isn.net/~jypsy/community.htm.

145 For discussions about benefits and dangers of realistic self-knowledge see Taylor and Brown 1988; Wilson and Dunn 2004.

146 The clinician Tony Attwood (1998) suggests we wait until children ask "why" they have difficulties.

147 This adevelopmental approach to autism contributes to a lack of knowledge about the earliest indicators of autism, and the late diagnosis of autism, which, as already mentioned, on average occurs at about six years (Filipek *et al.* 2000). Furthermore, not only does the DSM-IV not reflect any developmental aspect of autism, it also defines it through criteria appropriate only to early and middle childhood. The same is true for essentially adevelopmental psychological conceptions of autism. For example, Uta Frith's definition of autism—which tries to take its developmental aspects into account—states, "Its core features, present in different forms, at all stages of development and at all levels of ability, are impairments of socialization, communication, and imagination" (1991, p.2). But, although these impairments are the most pronounced in childhood autism, other more elementary impairments, such as lack of sensory-motor integration, might be better defining characteristics of autism at the earliest stages of development (for empirical support see Baranek 1999; Iwanaga, Kawasaki, and Tsuchida 2000).

148 *Defect* was a term used in Russia at that time to refer to any atypical development.

149 Autism often coexists with other developmental and/or psychiatric disorders (e.g., mental retardation, Attention Deficit Hyperactivity Disorder, obsessive-compulsive disorder, Tourette syndrome, depression, epilepsy, and anxiety).

150 We use the terms self-awareness, self-perception, self-understanding, and self-knowledge interchangeably to mean all aspects of self-understanding. For our purpose here, they refer to the awareness one has of one's body, actions, emotions, beliefs, knowledge, abilities, will, and so on; such awareness also refers to feelings of self-continuity (i.e., the link between one's past and possible/anticipated future experiences). Some of these aspects of self-understanding are also referred to in the psychological literature as se;f-consciousness, self-concept, self-esteem, or self-reflection.

151 It should be noted that the term "autistic" here refers to any of the diagnostic labels including Asperger's Disorder.

152 However, there have been recently some attempts to correct for this (Frith and Happé 1999; Hurlburt, Happé, and Frith 1994).

153 This claim is made in the face of autobiographical accounts by autistic persons (Bemporad 1979; Grandin and Scariano 1986; Miedzianik 1986). For example, Simon Baron-Cohen (1989c), one of the originators of the ToM deficit hypothesis in autism and one of the most active researchers and theorists in the field, wrote that autistic persons are incapable of self-reports.

154 Despite the supposed evolutionary importance of understanding others' minds—needed for survival purposes (Humphrey 1992)—from the perspective of living a good life, it is more important to know one's own strengths and limitations, needs and desires, and have a perspective on the possibilities for oneself.

155 Martin Buber distinguishes among three kinds of dialogue (1947, p.19): "There is genuine dialogue—no matter whether spoken or silent—where each of the participants really has in mind the other or others in their present and particular being and turns to them with the intention of establishing a living mutual relation between himself and them. There is technical dialogue, which is prompted solely by the

need of objective understanding. And there is monologue disguised as dialogue, in which two or men, meeting in space, speak each with himself in strangely tortuous and circuitous ways and yet imagine they have escaped the torment of being thrown back on their own resources."

156 A method suggested long ago by personality psychologists like Gordon Allport (1937) and George Kelly (1955).

157 This is a point already made by personality psychologists (Kelly 1955; Little 2000).

158 Here we adapt Temple Grandin's self-description as feeling "like an anthropologist on Mars" (Sacks 1996, p.259).

159 For discussion of some of these methodological issues, see Burack *et al.* 2002; Hobson 1991; Mervis and Klein-Tasman 2004; Mervis and Robinson 1999; Mottron 2004; Yule 1978. In fact, an entire recent issue of the *Journal of Autism and Developmental Disorders* (February, 2004) is devoted to problems associated with group studies of autism, particularly the issue of finding the appropriate matching groups needed to implement this kind of design, and statistical procedures involved in obtaining legitimate comparison between these groups.

160 The instruction was to describe himself to people who do not know anything about him—to describe what kind of person he is.

161 Contrast this to his do-not-disturb door sign from the time he was 12.

References

Adrien, J.L., Martineau, J. and Barthelemy, C. (1995) 'Disorders of regulation of cognitive activity in autistic children.' *Journal of Autism and Developmental Disorders 25*, 3, 249–263.

Akshoomoff, N., Pierce, K. and Courchesne, E. (2002) 'The neurobiological basis of autism from a developmental perspective.' *Development and Psychopathology 14*, 3, 613–634.

Allen, G., Buxton, R.B., Wong, E.C. and Courchesne, E. (1997) 'Attentional activation of the cerebellum independent of motor involvement.' *Science 275*, 5308, 1940–1943.

Allen, G. and Courchesne, E. (2001) 'Attention function and dysfunction in autism.' *Frontiers in Bioscience 6*, 105–119.

Allport, G.W. (1937) *Personality: A Psychological Interpretation.* New York: Henry Holt.

Allport, G.W. (1955) *Becoming: Basic Considerations for a Psychology of Personality.* New Haven, CN: Yale University Press.

Allport, G.W. (1961) *Pattern and Growth in Personality.* New York: Holt, Rinehart and Winston.

American Psychiatric Association (APA) (1994) *Diagnostic and Statistical Manual of Mental Disorders* (4th edn). Washington, DC: American Psychiatric Association.

American Psychiatric Association (APA) (2000) *Diagnostic and Statistical Manual of Mental Disorders* (DSM-IV-TR, 4th edn, text revision). Washington, DC: American Psychiatric Association.

Anderson, G.M. and Hoshino, Y. (1997) 'Neurochemical studies of autism.' In D.J. Cohen and F.R. Volkmar (eds) *Handbook of Autism and Pervasive Developmental Disorders* (2nd edn). New York: J. Wiley.

Asperger, H. (1979) 'Problems of infantile autism.' *Communication 13*, 45–52.

Asperger, H. (1944/1991) '"Autistic psychopathy" in childhood.' In U. Frith (ed.) *Autism and Asperger Syndrome.* Cambridge, UK: Cambridge University Press.

Attwood, T. (1998) *Asperger's Syndrome: A Guide for Parents and Professionals.* London: Jessica Kingsley Publishers.

Attwood, T. (2000) 'Strategies for improving the social integration of children with Asperger syndrome.' *Autism 4*, 1, 85–100.

autistics.org (1998) Institute for the Study of the Neurologically Typical. http://isnt.autistics.org.

Aylward, E.H., Minshew, N.J., Field, K., Sparks, B.F. and Singh, N. (2002) 'Effects of age on brain volume and head circumference in autism.' *Neurology 59*, 2, 175–183.

Aylward, E.H., Minshew, N.J., Goldstein, G., Honeycutt, N.A., Augustine, A.M., Yates, K.O., Barta, P.E. and Pearlson, G.D. (1999) 'MRI volumes of amygdala and hippocampus in non-mentally retarded autistic adolescents and adults.' *Neurology 53*, 9, 2145–2150.

Bacon, A.L., Fein, D., Morris, R., Waterhouse, L. and Allen, D. (1998) 'The responses of autistic children to the distress of others.' *Journal of Autism and Developmental Disorders 28*, 2, 129–142.

Bailey, A., Le Couteur, A., Gottesman, I., Bolton, P., Simonoff, E., Yuzda, E. and Rutter, M. (1995) 'Autism as a strongly genetic disorder: Evidence from a British twin study.' *Psychological Medicine 25*, 1, 63–77.

Bailey, A., Luthert, P., Dean, A., Harding, B., Janota, I., Montgomery, M., Rutter, M. and Lantos, P. (1998) 'A clinicopathological study of autism.' *Brain 121*, 5, 889–905.

Bailey, A., Phillips, W. and Rutter, M. (1996) 'Autism: Towards an integration of clinical, genetic, neuropsychological, and neurobiological perspectives.' *Journal of Child Psychology and Psychiatry 37*, 1, 89–126.

Bandura, A. (2001) 'Social cognitive theory: An agentic perspective.' *Annual Review of Psychology 52*, 1, 1–26.

Baranek, G.T. (1999) 'Autism during infancy: A retrospective video analysis of sensory-motor and social behaviors at 9–12 months of age.' *Journal of Autism and Developmental Disorders 29*, 3, 213–224.

Barnhill, G., Hagiwara, T., Myles, B.S. and Simpson, R.L. (2000) 'Asperger syndrome: A study of the cognitive profiles of 37 children and adolescents.' *Focus on Autism and Other Developmental Disabilities 15*, 3, 146–153.

Barnhill, G.P., Cook, K.T., Tebbenkamp, K. and Myles, B.S. (2002) 'The effectiveness of social skills intervention targeting nonverbal communication for adolescents with Asperger syndrome and related pervasive developmental delays.' *Focus on Autism and Other Developmental Disabilities 17*, 2, 112–118.

Baron-Cohen, S. (1989a) 'The autistic child's theory of mind: A case of specific developmental delay.' *Journal of Child Psychology and Psychiatry and Allied Disciplines 30*, 2, 285–297.

Baron-Cohen, S. (1989b) 'Are autistic children "behaviorists"? An examination of their mental-physical and appearance-reality distinctions.' *Journal of Autism and Developmental Disorders 19*, 4, 579–600.

Baron-Cohen, S. (1989c) 'Do autistic children have obsessions and compulsions?' *British Journal of Clinical Psychology 28*, 3, 193–200.

Baron-Cohen, S. (1991) 'Do people with autism understand what causes emotion?' *Child Development 62*, 2, 385–395.

Baron-Cohen, S. (1995) *Mindblindness: An Essay on Autism and Theory of Mind.* Cambridge, MA: MIT Press.

Baron-Cohen, S. (2000a) 'Is Asperger syndrome/high-functioning autism necessarily a disability?' *Development and Psychopathology 12*, 3, 489–500.

Baron-Cohen, S. (2000b) 'Autism: Deficits in folk psychology exist alongside superiority in folk physics.' In S. Baron-Cohen, H. Tager-Flusberg and D.J. Cohen (eds) *Understanding Other Minds: Perspectives from Developmental Cognitive Neuroscience.* Oxford: Oxford University Press.

Baron-Cohen, S. (2001) 'Theory of mind and autism: A review.' *International Review of Research in Mental Retardation 23*, 169–184.

Baron-Cohen, S., Cox, A., Baird, G., Swettenham, J., Nightingale, N., Morgan, K., Drew, A. and Charman, T. (1996) 'Psychological markers in the detection of autism in infancy in a large population.' *British Journal of Psychiatry 168*, 2, 158–163.

Baron-Cohen, S., Leslie, A.M. and Frith, U. (1985) 'Does the autistic child have a "theory of mind"?' *Cognition 21*, 1, 37–46.

Baron-Cohen, S., Leslie, A.M. and Frith, U. (1986) 'Mechanical, behavioural and intentional understanding of picture stories in autistic children.' *British Journal of Developmental Psychology 4*, 2, 113–125.

Baron-Cohen, S., Ring, H.A., Wheelwright, S., Bullmore, E.T., Brammer, M.J., Simmons, A. and Williams, S.C. (1999) 'Social intelligence in the normal and autistic brain: An fMRI study.' *European Journal of Neuroscience 11*, 6, 1891–1898.

Barron, J. and Barron, S. (2002) *There's a Boy in Here.* Arlington, TX: Future Hotizons.

Bauman, M.L. and Kemper, T.L. (1994) 'Neuroanatomic observations of the brain in autism.' In M.L. Bauman and T.L. Kemper (eds) *The Neurobiology of Autism.* Baltimore: The Johns Hopkins University Press.

Bemporad, J.R. (1979) 'Adult recollections of a formerly autistic child.' *Journal of Autism and Developmental Disorders 9*, 2, 179–197.

Bennetto, L., Pennington, B.F. and Rogers, S.J. (1996) 'Intact and impaired memory functions in autism.' *Child Development 67*, 4, 1816–1835.

Bernard, S., Enayati, A., Redwood, L., Roger, H. and Binstock, T. (2001) 'Autism: A novel form of mercury poisoning.' *Medical Hypotheses 56*, 4, 462–471.

Betancur, C., Corbex, M., Spielewoy, C., Philippe, A., Laplanche, J.L., Launay, J.M., Gillberg, C., Mouren-Simeoni, M.C., Hamon, M., Giros, B., Nosten-Bertrand, M., Leboyer, M. and the Paris Autism Research International Sibpair (PARIS) Study (2002) 'Serotonin transporter gene polymorphisms and hyperserotonemia in autistic disorder.' *Molecular Psychiatry 7*, 1, 67–71.

Blacher, J., Kraemer, B. and Schalow, M. (2003) 'Asperger syndrome and high functioning autism: Research concerns and emerging foci.' *Current Opinion in Psychiatry 16*, 5, 535–542.

Blair, R.J.R. (1999) 'Psychophysiological responsiveness to the distress of others in children with autism.' *Personality and Individual Differences 26*, 3, 477–485.

Blatt, G.J., Fitzgerald, C.M., Guptill, J.T., Booker, A.B., Kemper, T.L. and Bauman, M.L. (2001) 'Density and distribution of hippocampal neurotransmitter receptors in autism: An autoradiographic study.' *Journal of Autism and Developmental Disorders 31*, 6, 537–543.

Bleuler, E.P. (1916/1951) *Textbook of Psychiatry* (trans. A.A. Brill). New York: Dover.

Boddaert, N., Belin, P., Chabane, N., Poline, J.B., Barthelemy, C., Mouren-Simeoni, M.C., Brunelle, F., Samson, Y. and Zilbovicius, M. (2003) 'Perception of complex sounds: Abnormal pattern of cortical activation in autism.' *American Journal of Psychiatry 160,* 11, 2057–2060.

Boddaert, N. and Zilbovicius, M. (2002) 'Functional neuroimaging and childhood autism.' *Pediatric Radiology 32,* 1, 1–7.

Bogdan, R. and Biklen, S.K. (1998) *Qualitative Research for Education: An Introduction to Theory and Methods* (3rd edn). Boston, MA: Allyn and Bacon.

Bolton, P., Macdonald, H., Pickles, A. and Rios, P. (1994) 'A case-control family history study of autism.' *Journal of Child Psychology and Psychiatry and Allied Disciplines 35,* 5, 877–900.

Bolton, P.F., Murphy, M., Macdonald, H., Whitlock, B., Pickles, A. and Rutter, M. (1997) 'Obstetric complications in autism: Consequences or causes of the condition?' *Journal of the American Academy of Child and Adolescent Psychiatry 36,* 2, 272–281.

Bolton, P.F., Roobol, M., Allsopp, L. and Pickles, A. (2001) 'Association between idiopathic infantile macrocephaly and autism spectrum disorders.' *Lancet 358,* 9283, 726–727.

Bosch, G. (1962/1970) *Infantile Autism: A Clinical and Phenomenological-Anthropological Investigation Taking Language as the Guide* (trans. D. Jordan and I. Jordan). New York: Springer-Verlag.

Boucher, J. and Warrington, E.K. (1976) 'Memory deficits in early infantile autism: Some similarities to the amnesic syndrome.' *British Journal of Psychology 67,* 1, 73–87.

Bowler, D.M. (1992) '"Theory of mind" in Asperger's syndrome.' *Journal of Child Psychology and Psychiatry 33,* 5, 877–893.

Brambilla, P., Hardan, A., di Nemi, S.U., Perez, J., Soares, J.C. and Barale, F. (2003) 'Brain anatomy and development in autism: Review of structural MRI studies.' *Brain Research Bulletin 61,* 6, 557–569.

Broderick, C., Caswell, R., Gregory, S., Marzolini, S. and Wilson, O. (2002) '"Can I join the club?" A social integration scheme for adolescents with Asperger syndrome.' *Autism 6,* 4, 427–431.

Bronfenbrenner, U. (1979) *The Ecology of Human Development: Experiments by Nature and Design.* Cambridge, MA: Harvard University Press.

Bronfenbrenner, U. (1989) 'Ecological systems theory.' *Annals of Child Development 6,* 187–249.

Bruner, J. (1990) *Acts of Meaning.* Cambridge, MA: Harvard University Press.

Bruner, J. (1997) 'A narrative model of self-construction.' In J.G. Snodgrass and R.L. Thompson (eds) *The Self Across Psychology: Self-recognition, Self-awareness, and the Self Concept. Annals of the New York Academy of Sciences,* vol. 818. New York: New York Academy of Sciences.

Bruner, J.S. (2002) *Making Stories: Law, Literature, Life.* New York: Farrar, Straus, and Giroux.

Bryson, S.E., Wainwright-Sharp, J.A. and Smith, I.M. (1990) 'Autism: A developmental spatial neglect syndrome?' In J.T. Enns (ed.) *The Development of Attention: Research and Theory.* Amsterdam: Elsevier.

Buber, M. (1947) *Between Man and Man.* London: Kegan Paul.

Buber, M. (1965) *The Knowledge of Man.* New York: Harper and Row.

Burack, J.A. (1994) 'Selective attention deficits in persons with autism: Preliminary evidence of an inefficient attentional lens.' *Journal of Abnormal Psychology 103,* 3, 535–543.

Burack, J.A., Enns, J.T., Stauder, J.E.A., Mottron, L. and Randolph, B. (1997) 'Attention and autism: Behavioral and electrophysiological evidence.' In D.J. Cohen and F.R. Volkmar (eds) *Handbook of autism and pervasive developmental disorders* (2nd edn). New York: J. Wiley.

Burack, J.A., Iarocci, G., Bowler, D. and Mottron, L. (2002) 'Benefits and pitfalls in the merging of disciplines: The example of developmental psychopathology and the study of persons with autism.' *Development and Psychopathology 14,* 2, 225–237.

Capps, L., Sigman, M. and Mundy, P. (1994) 'Attachment security in children with autism.' *Development and Psychopathology 6,* 2, 249–261.

Capps, L., Sigman, M. and Yirmiya, N. (1995) 'Self-competence and emotional understanding in high-functioning children with autism. Special issue: Emotions in developmental psychopathology.' *Development and Psychopathology 7,* 1, 137–149.

Carpenter, A. (1992) 'Autistic adulthood: A challenging journey.' In E. Schopler and G.B. Mesibov (eds) *High-functioning Individuals with Autism.* New York: Plenum Press.

Cash, A.B. (1999) 'A profile of gifted individuals with autism: The twice-exceptional learner.' *Roeper Review 22,* 1, 22–27.

Castelli, F., Frith, C., Happé, F. and Frith, U. (2002) 'Autism, Asperger syndrome and brain mechanisms for the attribution of mental states to animated shapes.' *Brain 125,* pt 8, 1839–1849.

Cesaroni, L. and Garber, M. (1991) 'Exploring the experience of autism through firsthand accounts.' *Journal of Autism and Developmental Disorders 21,* 3, 303–313.

Chandler, M., Fritz, A.S. and Hala, S. (1989) 'Small-scale deceit: Deception as a marker of two-, three-, and four-year-olds' early theories of mind.' *Child Development 60*, 6, 1263–1277.

Charman, T., Swettenham, J., Baron-Cohen, S., Cox, A., Baird, G. and Drew, A. (1997) 'Infants with autism: An investigation of empathy, pretend play, joint attention, and imitation.' *Developmental Psychology 33*, 5, 781–789.

Chiron, C., Leboyer, M., Leon, F., Jambaque, I., Nuttin, C. and Syrota, A. (1995) 'SPECT of the brain in childhood autism: Evidence for a lack of normal hemispheric asymmetry.' *Developmental Medicine and Child Neurology 37*, 10, 849–860.

Chugani, D.C., Muzik, O., Behen, M., Rothermel, R., Janisse, J.J., Lee, J. and Chugani, H.T. (1999) 'Developmental changes in brain serotonin synthesis capacity in autistic and nonautistic children.' *Annals of Neurology 45*, 3, 287–295.

Chugani, D.C., Muzik, O., Rothermel, R., Behen, M., Chakraborty, P., Mangner, T., da Silva, E.A. and Chugani, H.T. (1997) 'Altered serotonin synthesis in the dentatothalamocortical pathway in autistic boys.' *Annals of Neurology 42*, 4, 666–669.

Cook, E.H. and Leventhal, B.L. (1996) 'The serotonin system in autism.' *Current Opinion in Pediatrics 8*, 4, 348–354.

Courchesne, E. (1997) 'Brainstem, cerebellar and limbic neuroanatomical abnormalities in autism.' *Current Opinion in Neurobiology 7*, 2, 269–278.

Courchesne, E., Carper, R. and Akshoomoff, N. (2003) 'Evidence of brain overgrowth in the first year of life in autism.' *Journal of the American Medical Association 290*, 3, 337–344.

Courchesne, E., Karns, C.M., Davis, H.R., Ziccardi, R., Carper, R.A., Tigue, Z.D., Chisum, H.J., Moses, P., Pierce, K., Lord, C., Lincoln, A.J., Pizzo, S., Schreibman, L., Haas, R.H., Akshoomoff, N.A. and Courchesne, R.Y. (2001) 'Unusual brain growth patterns in early life in patients with autistic disorder: An MRI study.' *Neurology 57*, 2, 245–254.

Courchesne, E., Lincoln, A.J., Kilman, B.A. and Galambos, R. (1985) 'Event-related brain potential correlates of the processing of novel visual and auditory information in autism.' *Journal of Autism and Developmental Disorders 15*, 1, 55–76.

Courchesne, E., Saitoh, O., Townsend, J.P., Yeung-Courchesne, R., Press, G.A., Lincoln, A.J., Haas, R.H. and Schriebman, L. (1994) 'Cerebellar hypoplasia and hyperplasia in infantile autism.' *Lancet 343*, 8888, 63–64.

Critchley, H.D., Daly, E.M., Bullmore, E.T., Williams, S.C., Van Amelsvoort, T., Robertson, D.M., Rowe, A., Phillips, M., McAlonan, G., Howlin, P. and Murphy, D.G. (2000) 'The functional neuroanatomy of social behaviour: Changes in cerebral blood flow when people with autistic disorder process facial expressions.' *Brain 123*, 11, 2203–2212.

Cytowic, R.E. (1993) *The Man who Tasted Shapes: A Bizarre Medical Mystery Offers Revolutionary Insights into Emotions, Reasoning and Consciousness.* New York: Jeremy P. Tarcher/Putnam.

Dahlgren, S.O. and Trillingsgaard, A. (1996) 'Theory of mind in non-retarded children with autism and Asperger's syndrome. A research note.' *Journal of Child Psychology and Psychiatry 37*, 6, 759–763.

Damon, W. and Hart, D. (1988) *Self-understanding in Childhood and Adolescence.* New York: Cambridge University Press.

Dawson, G. and Fernald, M. (1987) 'Perspective-taking ability and its relationship to the social behavior of autistic children.' *Journal of Autism and Developmental Disorders 17*, 4, 487–498.

Dawson, G. and McKissick, F.C. (1984) 'Self-recognition in autistic children.' *Journal of Autism and Developmental Disorders 14*, 4, 383–394.

Dawson, G., Webb, S., Schellenberg, G.D., Dager, S., Friedman, S., Aylward, E. and Richards, T. (2002) 'Defining the broader phenotype of autism: Genetic, brain, and behavioral perspectives.' *Development and Psychopathology 14*, 3, 581–611.

Dawson, M. (2003) *NO AUTISTICS ALLOWED: Autism Society Canada Speaks For Itself: AN OPEN LETTER*, retrieved October from http://www.sentex.net/~nexus23/naa_02.html.

DeStefano, F., Bhasin, T.K., Thompson, W.W., Yeargin-Allsopp, M. and Boyle, C. (2004) 'Age at first measles-mumps-rubella vaccination in children with autism and school-matched control subjects: A population-based study in metropolitan Atlanta.' *Pediatrics 113*, 2, 259–266.

Dewey, M. (1991) 'Living with Asperger's syndrome.' In U. Frith (ed.) *Autism and Asperger Syndrome.* Cambridge, UK: Cambridge University Press.

Dissanayake, C. and Sigman, M. (2001) 'Attachment and emotional responsiveness in children with autism.' *International Review of Research in Mental Retardation 23*, 239–266.

Donchin, E. (1981) 'Surprise!...Surprise?' *Psychophysiology 18*, 5, 493–513.

Dunn, W., Saiter, J. and Rinner, L. (2002) 'Asperger syndrome and sensory processing: A conceptual model and guidance for intervention planning.' *Focus on Autism and Other Developmental Disabilities 17*, 3, 172–185.

Egaas, B., Courchesne, E. and Saitoh, O. (1995) 'Reduced size of corpus callosum in autism.' *Archives of Neurology 52*, 8, 794–801.

Ehlers, S., Nyden, A., Gillberg, C., Sandberg, A.D., Dahlgren, S.O., Hjelmquist, E. and Oden, A. (1997) 'Asperger syndrome, autism and attention disorders: A comparative study of the cognitive profiles of 120 children.' *Journal of Child Psychology and Psychiatry 38*, 2, 207–217.

Eisenmajer, R., Prior, M., Leekam, S., Wing, L., Gould, J., Welham, M. and Ong, B. (1996) 'Comparison of clinical symptoms in autism and Asperger's disorder.' *Journal of the American Academy of Child and Adolescent Psychiatry 35*, 11, 1523–1531.

Elliott, G.R. and Ciaranello, R.D. (1987) 'Neurochemical hypotheses of childhood psychoses.' In E. Schopler and G.B. Mesibov (eds) *Neurobiological Issues in Autism.* New York: Plenum Press.

Ernst, M., Zametkin, A.J., Matochik, J.A., Pascualvaca, D. and Cohen, R.M. (1997) 'Low medial prefrontal dopaminergic activity in autistic children.' *Lancet 350*, 9078, 638.

Farrant, A., Blades, M. and Boucher, J. (1998) 'Source monitoring by children with autism.' *Journal of Autism and Developmental Disorders 28*, 1, 43–50.

Fatemi, S.H., Halt, A.R., Stary, J.M., Kanodia, R., Schulz, S.C. and Realmuto, G.R. (2002) 'Glutamic acid decarboxylase 65 and 67 kDa proteins are reduced in autistic parietal and cerebellar cortices.' *Biological Psychiatry 52*, 8, 805–810.

Fecteau, S., Mottron, L., Berthiaume, C. and Burack, J.A. (2003) 'Developmental changes of autistic symptoms.' *Autism 7*, 3, 255–268.

Ferrari, M. (2003) 'Educating selves to be creative and wise.' In M. Ferrari (ed.) *Beyond Knowledge: Non-cognitive Aspects of Developing High Ability.* Mahwah, NJ: Lawrence Erlbaum.

Ferrari, M. and Mahalingam, R. (1998) 'Personal cognitive development and its implications for teaching and learning.' *Educational Psychologist 33*, 1, 35–44.

Filipek, P.A., Accardo, P.J., Ashwal, S., Baranek, G.T., Cook, E.H., Jr., Dawson, G., Gordon, B., Gravel, J.S., Johnson, C.P., Kallen, R.J., Levy, S.E., Minshew, N.J., Ozonoff, S., Prizant, B.M., Rapin, I., Rogers, S.J., Stone, W.L., Teplin, S.W., Tuchman, R.F. and Volkmar, F.R. (2000) 'Practice parameter: Screening and diagnosis of autism: Report of the Quality Standards Subcommittee of the American Academy of Neurology and the Child Neurology Society.' *Neurology 55*, 4, 468–479.

Flavell, J.H. (1999) 'Cognitive development: Children's knowledge about the mind.' *Annual Review of Psychology 50*, 21–45.

Fogel, A. (1990) 'The process of developmental change in infant communicative action: Using dynamic systems theory to study individual ontogenies.' In J. Colombo and J. Fagen (eds) *Individual Differences in Infancy: Reliability, Stability, Prediction.* Hillsdale, NJ: Lawrence Erlbaum.

Fogel, A. (1993) *Developing Through Relationships: Origins of Communication, Self, and Culture.* Chicago, IL: University of Chicago Press.

Folstein, S.E. and Rosen-Sheidley, B. (2001) 'Genetics of autism: Complex aetiology for a heterogeneous disorder.' *Nature Reviews Genetics 2*, 12, 943–955.

Folstein, S.E. and Santangelo, S.L. (2000) 'Does Asperger syndrome aggregate in families?' In A. Klin, F.R. Volkmar and S.S. Sparrow (eds) *Asperger Syndrome.* New York: Guilford Press.

Freeman, M. (2001) 'From substance to story: Narrative, identity, and the reconstruction of the self.' In J. Brockmeier and D.A. Carbaugh (eds) *Narrative and Identity: Studies in Autobiography, Self and Culture.* Amsterdam, Netherlands: John Benjamins.

Freeman, M. and Brockmeier, J. (2001) 'Narrative integrity: Autobiographical identity and the meaning of the "good life".' In J. Brockmeier and D.A. Carbaugh (eds) *Narrative and Identity: Studies in Autobiography, Self and Culture.* Amsterdam, Netherlands: John Benjamins.

Frith, U. (1989) *Autism: Explaining the Enigma.* Oxford: Blackwell.

Frith, U. (1991) 'Asperger and his syndrome.' In U. Frith (ed.) *Autism and Asperger Syndrome.* Cambridge, UK: Cambridge University Press.

Frith, U. (2001) 'Mind blindness and the brain in autism.' *Neuron 32*, 6, 969–979.

Frith, U. and Happé, F. (1994) 'Autism: Beyond "theory of mind".' *Cognition 50*, 1–3, 115–132.

Frith, U. and Happé, F. (1999) 'Theory of mind and self-consciousness: What is it like to be autistic?' *Mind and Language 14*, 1, 1–22.

Gaffney, G.R., Kuperman, S., Tsai, L.Y. and Minchin, S. (1989) 'Forebrain structure in infantile autism.' *Journal of the American Academy of Child and Adolescent Psychiatry 28*, 4, 534–537.

Gardner, H. (1993) *Multiple Intelligences: The Theory in Practice.* New York: Basic Books.

Gardner, H. (1997) *Extraordinary Minds: Portraits of Exceptional Individuals and an Examination of our Extraordinariness.* New York: Basic Books.

Gardner, H. (1998) 'A multiplicity of intelligences.' *Scientific American 9*, 4, 18–23.

Gardner, H. (2002) 'Learning from extraordinary minds.' In M. Ferrari (ed.) *The Pursuit of Excellence through Education.* Mahwah, NJ: Lawrence Erlbaum.

Gauthier, I. and Tarr, M.J. (1997) 'Becoming a "Greeble" expert: Exploring mechanisms for face recognition.' *Vision Research 37*, 12, 1673–1682.

George, M.S., Costa, D.C., Kouris, K., Ring, H.A. and Ell, P.J. (1992) 'Cerebral blood flow abnormalities in adults with infantile autism.' *The Journal of Nervous and Mental Disease 180*, 7, 413–417.

Ghaziuddin, M. (1996) 'Pedantic speaking style differentiates Asperger syndrome from high-functioning autism.' *Journal of Autism and Developmental Disorders 26*, 6, 585–595.

Ghaziuddin, M., Butler, E., Tsai, L. and Ghaziuddin, N. (1994) 'Is clumsiness a marker for Asperger syndrome?' *Journal of Intellectual Disability Research 38*, 5, 519–527.

Gilchrist, A., Green, J., Cox, A., Burton, D., Rutter, M. and Le Couteur, A. (2001) 'Development and current functioning in adolescents with Asperger syndrome: A comparative study.' *Journal of Child Psychology and Psychiatry and Allied Disciplines 42*, 2, 227–240.

Gillberg, C. (1989) 'Asperger syndrome in 23 Swedish children.' *Developmental Medicine and Child Neurology 31*, 4, 520–531.

Gillberg, C. (1990) 'Autism and pervasive developmental disorders.' *Journal of Child Psychology and Psychiatry and Allied Disciplines 31*, 1, 99–119.

Gillberg, C. (1991) 'Clinical and neurobiological aspects of Asperger syndrome in six family studies.' In U. Frith (ed.) *Autism and Asperger Syndrome.* New York: Cambridge University Press.

Gillberg, C. (1992) 'Autism and autistic-like conditions: Subclasses among disorders of empathy. The Emanuel Miller Memorial Lecture 1991.' *Journal of Child Psychology and Psychiatry 33*, 5, 813–842.

Gillberg, C. (1998) 'Chromosomal disorders and autism.' *Journal of Autism and Developmental Disorders 28*, 5, 415–425.

Gillberg, C. (2002) *A Guide to Asperger Syndrome.* Cambridge, UK: Cambridge University Press.

Gillberg, C. and Svennerholm, L. (1987) 'CSF monoamines in autistic syndromes and other pervasive developmental disorders of early childhood.' *British Journal of Psychiatry 151*, 89–94.

Gillberg, I.C., Bjure, J., Uvebrant, P., Vestergren, E. and Gillberg, C. (1993) 'SPECT in 31 children and adolescents with autism and autistic-like conditions.' *European Child and Adolescent Psychiatry 2*, 50–59.

Gloor, P. (1997) *The Temporal Lobe and Limbic System.* New York: Oxford University Press.

Goodman, N. (1978) *Ways of Worldmaking.* Indianapolis: Hackett.

Grandin, T. (1984) 'My experiences as an autistic-child and review of selected literature.' *Journal of Orthomolecular Psychiatry 13*, 3, 144–174.

Grandin, T. (1992) 'An inside view of autism.' In E. Schopler and G.B. Mesibov (eds) *High-functioning Individuals with Autism.* New York: Plenum Press.

Grandin, T. (1995a) 'How people with autism think.' In E. Schopler and G.B. Mesibov (eds) *Learning and Cognition in Autism.* New York: Plenum Press.

Grandin, T. (1995b) *Thinking in Pictures: And Other Reports from my Life with Autism.* New York: Doubleday.

Grandin, T. (1997) 'A personal perspective on autism.' In D.J. Cohen and F.R. Volkmar (eds) *Handbook of Autism and Pervasive Developmental Disorders* (2nd edn). New York: J. Wiley.

Grandin, T. (2000) 'Autistic emotions.' Retrieved January 10, 2002 from the world wide web: http://www.autism-society.org/packages/aspergers_emotions.html.

Grandin, T. and Scariano, M. (1986) *Emergence: Labeled Autistic.* New York: Warner Books.

Granic, I. and Hollenstein, T. (2003) 'Dynamic systems methods for models of developmental psychopathology.' *Development and Psychopathology 15*, 3, 641–669.

Gray, C. (1993) *Taming the Recess Jungle.* Arlington, TX: Future Horizons.

Gray, C. (1994) *Comic Strip Conversations.* Arlington, TX: Future Horizons.

Gray, C. (1998) 'Social stories and comic strip conversations with students with Asperger syndrome and high-functioning autism.' In E. Schopler, G.B. Mesibov and L.J. Kunce (eds) *Asperger syndrome or high functioning autism?* New York: Plenum Press.

Gray, C. and Attwood, T. (1999) 'The discovery of "Aspie" criteria by Attwood and Gray.' *The Morning News 11* [quarterly publication of Jemison Public Schools, Jemison, MI].

Green, D., Baird, G., Barnett, A.L., Henderson, L., Huber, J. and Henderson, S.E. (2002) 'The severity and nature of motor impairment in Asperger's syndrome: A comparison with specific developmental disorder of motor function.' *Journal of Child Psychology and Psychiatry and Allied Disciplines 43*, 5, 655–668.

Green, J., Gilchrist, A., Burton, D. and Cox, A. (2000) 'Social and psychiatric functioning in adolescents with Asperger syndrome compared with conduct disorder.' *Journal of Autism and Developmental Disorders 30*, 4, 279–293.

Green, L., Fein, D., Joy, S. and Waterhouse, L. (1995) 'Cognitive functioning in autism: An overview.' In E. Schopler and G.B. Mesibov (eds) *Learning and Cognition in Autism.* New York: Plenum Press.

Green, L., Fein, D., Modahl, C., Feinstein, C., Waterhouse, L. and Morris, M. (2001) 'Oxytocin and autistic disorder: Alterations in peptide forms.' *Biological Psychiatry 50*, 8, 609–613.

Gunter, H.L., Ghaziuddin, M. and Ellis, H.D. (2002) 'Asperger syndrome: Tests of right hemisphere functioning and interhemispheric communication.' *Journal of Autism and Developmental Disorders 32*, 4, 263–281.

Hagger, M.S., Biddle, S.J.H., Chow, E.W., Stambulova, N. and Kavussanu, M. (2003) 'Physical self-perceptions in adolescence: Generalizability of a hierarchical multidimensional model across three cultures.' *Journal of Cross-Cultural Psychology 34*, 6, 611–628.

Hanley, H.G., Stahl, S.M. and Freedman, D.X. (1977) 'Hyperserotonemia and amine metabolites in autistic and retarded children.' *Archives of General Psychiatry 34*, 5, 521–531.

Happé, F. (1991) 'The autobiographical writings of three Asperger syndrome adults: Problems of interpretation and implications for theory.' In U. Frith (ed.) *Autism and Asperger Syndrome.* Cambridge, UK: Cambridge University Press.

Happé, F. (1994a) *Autism: An Introduction to Psychological Theory.* Cambridge, MA: Harvard University Press.

Happé, F. (1994b) 'Wechsler IQ profile and theory of mind in autism: A research note.' *Journal of Child Psychology and Psychiatry 35*, 8, 1461–1471.

Happé, F. (1999a) 'Autism: Cognitive deficit or cognitive style?' *Trends in Cognitive Sciences 3*, 6, 216–222.

Happé, F. (1999b) 'Understanding assets and deficits in autism: Why success is more interesting than failure.' *Psychologist 12*, 11, 540–546.

Happé, F. (2003) 'Theory of mind and the self.' *Annals of the New York Academy of Sciences 1001*, 1, 134–144.

Happé, F., Ehlers, S., Fletcher, P., Frith, U., Johansson, M., Gillberg, C., Dolan, R., Frackowiak, R. and Frith, C. (1996) '"Theory of mind" in the brain. Evidence from a PET scan study of Asperger syndrome.' *NeuroReport 8*, 1, 197–201.

Hardan, A.Y., Minshew, N.J. and Keshavan, M.S. (2000) 'Corpus callosum size in autism.' *Neurology 55*, 7, 1033–1036.

Harré, R. (1983) *Personal Being: A Theory for Individual Psychology.* Cambridge, MA: Harvard University Press.

Harter, S. (1985) *Manual of the Self-Perception Profile for Children.* Denver, CO: University of Denver.

Harter, S. (1998) 'The development of self-representations.' In W. Damon (series ed.) and N. Eisenberg (vol. ed.) *Handbook of Child Psychology: Vol. 3. Social, Emotional, and Personality Development* (5th edn). New York: Wiley.

Harter, S. (1999) *The Construction of the Self: A Developmental Perspective.* New York: Guilford Press.

Hashimoto, T., Tayama, M., Miyazaki, M., Sakurama, N., Yoshimoto, T., Murakawa, K. and Kuroda, Y. (1992) 'Reduced brainstem size in children with autism.' *Brain and Development 14*, 2, 94–97.

Hauck, M., Fein, D., Waterhouse, L. and Feinstein, C. (1995) 'Social initiations by autistic children to adults and other children.' *Journal of Autism and Developmental Disorders 25*, 6, 579–595.

Haznedar, M.M., Buchsbaum, M.S., Wei, T.C., Hof, P.R., Cartwright, C., Bienstock, C.A. and Hollander, E. (2000) 'Limbic circuitry in patients with autism spectrum disorders studied with positron emission tomography and magnetic resonance imaging.' *American Journal of Psychiatry 157*, 12, 1994–2001.

Hérault, J., Petit, E., Martineau, J., Cherpi, C., Perrot, A., Barthelemy, C., Lelord, G. and Muh, J.P. (1996) 'Serotonin and autism: Biochemical and molecular biology features.' *Psychiatry Research 65*, 1, 33–43.

Hermelin, B. and O'Connor, N. (1964) 'Effects of sensory input and sensory dominance on severely disturbed autistic children and on subnormal controls.' *British Journal of Psychology 55*, 2, 201–206.

Hermelin, B. and O'Connor, N. (1970) *Psychological Experiments with Autistic Children.* Oxford: Pergamon Press.

Hill, E.L. (2004) 'Executive dysfunction in autism.' *Trends in Cognitive Sciences 8*, 1, 26–32.

Hill, E.L. and Russell, J. (2002) 'Action memory and self-monitoring in children with autism: Self versus other.' *Infant and Child Development 11*, 2, 159–170.
Hobson, R.P. (1986) 'The autistic child's appraisal of expressions of emotion.' *Journal of Child Psychology and Psychiatry 27*, 3, 321–342.
Hobson, R.P. (1989) 'Beyond cognition: A theory of autism.' In G. Dawson (ed.) *Autism: Nature, Diagnosis, and Treatment.* New York: Guilford Press.
Hobson, R.P. (1991) 'Methodological issues for experiments on autistic individuals' perception and understanding of emotion.' *Journal of Child Psychology and Psychiatry 32*, 7, 1135–1158.
Hobson, R.P. (1993) *Autism and the Development of Mind.* Hove, Sussex: Lawrence Erlbaum.
Hobson, R.P. and Lee, A. (1999) 'Imitation and identification in autism.' *Journal of Child Psychology and Psychiatry 40*, 4, 649–659.
Hobson, R.P., Ouston, J. and Lee, A. (1989) 'Naming emotion in faces and voices: Abilities and disabilities in autism and mental retardation.' *British Journal of Developmental Psychology 7*, 3, 237–250.
Hodgdon, L.Q. (1995) 'Solving social-behavioral problems through the use of visually supported communication.' In K.A. Quill (ed.) *Teaching Children with Autism: Strategies to Enhance Communication and Socialization.* New York: Delmar Publishers.
Holliday Willey, L. (1999) *Pretending to be Normal: Living with Asperger's Syndrome.* London: Jessica Kingsley Publishers.
Howard, M.A., Cowell, P.E., Boucher, J., Broks, P., Mayes, A., Farrant, A. and Roberts, N. (2000) 'Convergent neuroanatomical and behavioural evidence of an amygdala hypothesis of autism.' *NeuroReport 11*, 13, 2931–2935.
Howlin, P. (1998) *Children with Autism and Asperger Syndrome: A Guide for Practitioners and Carers.* Chichester: J. Wiley.
Howlin, P. (2003) 'Outcome in high-functioning adults with autism with and without early language delays: Implications for the differentiation between autism and Asperger syndrome.' *Journal of Autism and Developmental Disorders 33*, 1, 3–13.
Howlin, P., Baron-Cohen, S. and Hadwin, J. (1999) *Teaching Children with Autism to Mind-read: A Practical Guide for Teachers and Parents.* Chichester: J. Wiley.
Howlin, P., Goode, S., Hutton, J. and Rutter, M. (2004) 'Adult outcome for children with autism.' *Journal of Child Psychology and Psychiatry 45*, 2, 212–229.
Hubl, D., Bolte, S., Feineis-Matthews, S., Lanfermann, H., Federspiel, A., Strik, W., Poustka, F. and Dierks, T. (2003) 'Functional imbalance of visual pathways indicates alternative face processing strategies in autism.' *Neurology 61*, 9, 1232–1237.
Humphrey, N. (1992) *A History of the Mind: Evolution and the Birth of Consciousness.* New York: Simon and Schuster.
Hurlburt, R.T., Happé, F. and Frith, U. (1994) 'Sampling the form of inner experience in three adults with Asperger syndrome.' *Psychological Medicine 24*, 2, 385–395.
Hurlbutt, K. and Chalmers, L. (2002) 'Adults with autism speak out: Perceptions of their life experiences.' *Focus on Autism and Other Developmental Disabilities 17*, 2, 103–111.
International Molecular Genetic Study of Autism Consortium (IMGSAC) (2001) 'A genomewide screen for autism: Strong evidence for linkage to chromosomes 2q, 7q, and 16p.' *American Journal of Human Genetics 69*, 3, 570–581.
Iwanaga, R., Kawasaki, C. and Tsuchida, R. (2000) 'Brief report: Comparison of sensory-motor and cognitive function between autism and Asperger syndrome in preschool children.' *Journal of Autism and Developmental Disorders 30*, 2, 169–174.
Jackson, L. (2002) *Freaks, Geeks and Asperger Syndrome: A User Guide to Adolescence.* London: Jessica Kingsley Publishers.
Jacobs, B.L. and Azmitia, E.C. (1992) 'Structure and function of the brain serotonin system.' *Physiological Reviews 72*, 1, 165–229.
James, W. (1890) *The Principles of Psychology.* Cambridge, MA: Harvard University Press.
James, W. (1902) *The Varieties of Religious Experience: A Study in Human Nature.* London: Longmans Green.
Jansson-Verkasalo, E., Ceponiene, R., Kielinen, M., Suominen, K., Jantti, V., Linna, S.-L., Moilanen, I. and Naatanen, R. (2003) 'Deficient auditory processing in children with Asperger syndrome, as indexed by event-related potentials.' *Neuroscience Letters 338*, 3, 197–200.
Jolliffe, T., Lansdown, R. and Robinson, C. (1992) 'Autism: A personal account.' *Communication 26*, 12–19.

Kamps, D., Royer, J., Dugan, E., Kravits, T., Gonzalez Lopez, A., Garcia, J., Carnazzo, K., Morrison, L. and Kane, L.G. (2002) 'Peer training to facilitate social interaction for elementary students with autism and their peers.' *Exceptional Children 68*, 2, 173–187.

Kane, R.C. (2004) 'A possible association between fetal/neonatal exposure to radiofrequency electromagnetic radiation and the increased incidence of Autism Spectrum Disorders (ASD).' *Medical Hypotheses 62*, 2, 195–197.

Kanner, L. (1943) 'Autistic disturbances of affective contact.' *Nervous Child 2*, 217–250.

Kanner, L. (1971) 'Follow-up study of eleven autistic children originally reported in 1943.' *Journal of Autism and Childhood Schizophrenia 1*, 2, 119–145.

Kanner, L. (1973) 'How far can autistic children go in matters of social adaptation?' In L. Kanner (ed.) *Childhood Psychosis: Initial Studies and New Insights.* Washington: V.H. Winston.

Karmiloff-Smith, A. (1998) 'Development itself is the key to understanding developmental disorders.' *Trends in Cognitive Sciences 2*, 10, 389–398.

Kelly, G.A. (1955) *The Psychology of Personal Constructs.* New York: Norton.

Kim, J.A., Szatmari, P., Bryson, S.E., Streiner, D.L. and Wilson, F.J. (2000) 'The prevalence of anxiety and mood problems among children with autism and Asperger syndrome.' *Autism 4*, 2, 117–132.

Klin, A. and Volkmar, F.R. (2000) 'Treatment and intervention guidelines for individuals with Asperger syndrome.' In A. Klin, F.R. Volkmar and S.S. Sparrow (eds) *Asperger Syndrome.* New York: Guilford Press.

Klin, A., Volkmar, F.R., Sparrow, S.S., Cicchetti, D.V. and Rourke, B.P. (1995) 'Validity and neuropsychological characterization of Asperger syndrome: Convergence with nonverbal learning disabilities syndrome.' *Journal of Child Psychology and Psychiatry 36*, 7, 1127–1140.

Koenig, K., Tsatsanis, K.D. and Volkmar, F.R. (2001) 'Neurobiology and genetics of autism: A developmental perspective.' In J.A. Burack, T. Charman, N. Yirmiya and P.R. Zelazo (eds) *The Development of Autism: Perspectives from Theory and Research.* Mahwah, NJ: Lawrence Erlbaum.

Krause, I., He, X.S., Gershwin, M.E. and Shoenfeld, Y. (2002) 'Brief report: Immune factors in autism: A critical review.' *Journal of Autism and Developmental Disorders 32*, 4, 337–345.

Kunce, L. and Mesibov, G.B. (1998) 'Educational approaches to high-functioning autism and Asperger syndrome.' In E. Schopler, G.B. Mesibov and L.J. Kunce (eds) *Asperger Syndrome or High Functioning Autism?* New York: Plenum Press.

Kundera, M. (1991) *Immortality.* London: Faber and Faber.

Kvale, S. (1996) *InterViews: An Introduction to Qualitative Research Interviewing.* Thousand Oaks, CA: Sage.

Lainhart, J.E., Piven, J., Wzorek, M., Landa, R., Santangelo, S.L., Coon, H. and Folstein, S.E. (1997) 'Macrocephaly in children and adults with autism.' *Journal of the American Academy of Child and Adolescent Psychiatry 36*, 2, 282–290.

Lamb, J.A., Moore, J., Bailey, A. and Monaco, A.P. (2000) 'Autism: Recent molecular genetic advances.' *Human Molecular Genetics 9*, 6, 861–868.

Le Couteur, A., Bailey, A., Goode, S., Pickles, A., Robertson, S., Gottesman, I. and Rutter, M. (1996) 'A broader phenotype of autism: The clinical spectrum in twins.' *Journal of Child Psychology and Psychiatry 37*, 7, 785–801.

Lee, A. and Hobson, R.P. (1998) 'On developing self-concepts: A controlled study of children and adolescents with autism.' *Journal of Child Psychology and Psychiatry and Allied Disciplines 39*, 8, 1131–1144.

Leekam, S.R., Lopez, B. and Moore, C. (2000) 'Attention and joint attention in preschool children with autism.' *Developmental Psychology 36*, 2, 261–273.

Lewin, K. (1931/1935) *A Dynamic Theory of Personality: Selected Papers.* New York: McGraw-Hill (originally published in the *Journal of General Psychology 5* (1931), 141–177).

Lewin, K. (1951) *Field Theory in Social Science: Selected Theoretical Papers* (ed. D. Cartwright). New York: Harper and Row.

Lewis, M.D. and Ferrari, M. (2001) 'Cognitive-emotional self-organization in personality development and personal identity.' In H.A. Bosma and E.S. Kunnen (eds) *Identity and Emotions: A Self-organizational Perspective.* Cambridge, MA: Cambridge University Press.

Lincoln, A.J., Allen, M.H. and Kilman, A. (1995) 'The assessment and interpretation of intellectual abilities in people with autism.' In E. Schopler and G.B. Mesibov (eds) *Learning and Cognition in Autism.* New York: Plenum Press.

Lincoln, A., Courchesne, E., Allen, M., Hanson, E. and Ene, M. (1998) 'Neurobiology of Asperger syndrome: Seven case studies and quantitative magnetic resonance imaging findings.' In E. Schopler,

G.B. Mesibov and L.J. Kunce (eds) *Asperger Syndrome or High-functioning Autism?* New York: Plenum Press.

Lincoln, A.J., Courchesne, E., Harms, L. and Allen, M. (1993) 'Contextual probability evaluation in autistic, receptive developmental language disorder, and control children: Event-related brain potential evidence.' *Journal of Autism and Developmental Disorders 23*, 1, 37–58.

Liss, M., Fein, D., Allen, D., Dunn, M., Feinstein, C., Morris, R., Waterhouse, L. and Rapin, I. (2001) 'Executive functioning in high-functioning children with autism.' *Journal of Child Psychology and Psychiatry 42*, 2, 261–270.

Little, B.R. (2000) 'Persons, contexts, and personal projects: Assumptive themes of a methodological transactionalism.' In S. Wapner (ed.) *Theoretical Perspectives in Environment Behavior Research: Underlying Assumptions, Research Problems, and Methodologies.* Dordrecht, Netherlands: Kluwer Academic Publishers.

Little, C. (2002) 'Which is it? Asperger's syndrome or giftedness? Defining the differences.' *Gifted Child Today 25*, 1, 58–63.

Little, L. (2001) 'Peer victimization of children with Asperger spectrum disorders.' *Journal of the American Academy of Child and Adolescent Psychiatry 40*, 9, 995–996.

Locke, J. (1960/1997) *An Essay Concerning Human Understanding* (6th, revised edn). London: Penguin Books.

Lord, C. (1995) 'Follow-up of two-year-olds referred for possible autism.' *Journal of Child Psychology and Psychiatry 36*, 8, 1365–1382.

Lord, C., Cook, E.H., Leventhal, B.L. and Amaral, D.G. (2000) 'Autism spectrum disorders.' *Neuron 28*, 2, 355–363.

Lord, C. and Paul, R. (1997) 'Language and communication in autism.' In D.J. Cohen and F.R. Volkmar (eds) *Handbook of Autism and Pervasive Developmental Disorders* (2nd edn). New York: J. Wiley.

Lotspeich, L.J., Kwon, H., Schumann, C., Fryer, S., Goodlin-Jones, B.L., Buonocore, M.H., Lammers, C., Amaral, D. and Reiss, A. (2004) 'Investigation of neuroanatomical differences between autism and Asperger syndrome.' *Archives of General Psychiatry 61*, 3, 291–298.

Lovaas, O.I., Koegel, R.L. and Schreibman, L. (1979) 'Stimulus overselectivity in autism: A review of research.' *Psychological Bulletin 86*, 6, 1236–1254.

Loveland, K.A. and Landry, S.H. (1986) 'Joint attention and language in autism and developmental language delay.' *Journal of Autism and Developmental Disorders 16*, 3, 335–349.

Lucey, J.V., Costa, D.C., Busatto, G., Pilowsky, L.S., Marks, I.M., Ell, P.J. and Kerwin, R.W. (1997) 'Caudate regional cerebral blood flow in obsessive-compulsive disorder, panic disorder and healthy controls on single photon emission computerised tomography.' *Psychiatry Research 74*, 1, 25–33.

Luria, A.R. (1968) *The Mind of a Mnemonist.* New York: Basic Books.

Luria, A.R. (1972) *The Man with a Shattered World: The History of a Brain Wound* (trans. L. Solotaroff). New York: Basic Books.

Luria, A.R. (1979) *The Making of Mind: A Personal Account of Soviet Psychology* (trans. M. Cole). Cambridge, MA: Harvard University Press.

MacIntyre, A.C. (1981) *After Virtue: A Study in Moral Theory.* Notre Dame, IN: University of Notre Dame Press.

Manjiviona, J. and Prior, M. (1995) 'Comparison of Asperger syndrome and high-functioning autistic children on a test of motor impairment.' *Journal of Autism and Developmental Disorders 25*, 1, 23–39.

Manjiviona, J. and Prior, M. (1999) 'Neuropsychological profiles of children with Asperger syndrome and autism.' *Autism 3*, 4, 327–356.

Markus, H. and Nurius, P. (1986) 'Possible selves.' *American Psychologist 41*, 9, 954–969.

Markus, H. and Kitayama, S. (1991) 'Culture and the self: Implications for cognition, emotion, and motivation.' *Psychological Review 98*, 2, 224–253.

Mayes, S.D., Calhoun, S.L. and Crites, D.L. (2001) 'Does DSM-IV Asperger's disorder exist?' *Journal of Abnormal Child Psychology 29*, 3, 263–271.

McAdams, D.P. (1990) 'Unity and purpose in human lives: The emergence of identity as a life story.' In A.I. Rabin, R.A. Zucker, R.A. Emmons and F. Susan (eds) *Studying Persons and Lives.* New York: Springer Publishing.

McAdams, D.P. (1993) *The Stories We Live By: Personal Myths and the Making of the Self.* New York: Guilford Press.

McAdams, D.P. (1995) 'What do we know when we know a person?' *Journal of Personality 63*, 3, 365–397.

McDougle, C.J. and Posey, D.M.D. (2002) 'Genetics of childhood disorders: XLIV. Autism, Part 3: Psychopharmacology of autism.' *Journal of the American Academy of Child and Adolescent Psychiatry 41*, 11, 1380–1383.

McKelvey, J.R., Lambert, R., Mottron, L. and Shevell, M.I. (1995) 'Right-hemisphere dysfunction in Asperger's syndrome.' *Journal of Child Neurology 10*, 4, 310–314.

Meltzoff, A. and Gopnik, A. (1993) 'The role of imitation in understanding persons and developing a Theory of Mind.' In S. Baron-Cohen, H. Tager-Flusberg and D.J. Cohen (eds) *Understanding Other Minds: Perspectives from Autism.* Oxford: Oxford University Press.

Mercier, C., Mottron, L. and Belleville, S. (2000) 'A psychosocial study on restricted interests in high-functioning persons with pervasive developmental disorders.' *Autism 4*, 4, 406–425.

Mervis, C.B. and Klein-Tasman, B.P. (2004) 'Methodological issues in group-matching designs: A levels for control variable comparisons and measurement characteristics of control and target variables.' *Journal of Autism and Developmental Disorders 34*, 1, 7–17.

Mervis, C.B. and Robinson, B.F. (1999) 'Methodological issues in cross-syndrome comparisons: Matching procedures, sensitivity (Se), and specificity (Sp).' *Monographs of the Society for Research in Child Development 64*, 1, 115–130.

Miedzianik, D.C. (1986) *My Autobiography.* Nottingham: University of Nottingham.

Miller, J.N. and Ozonoff, S. (1997) 'Did Asperger's cases have Asperger disorder? A research note.' *Journal of Child Psychology and Psychiatry 38*, 2, 247–251.

Miller, J.N. and Ozonoff, S. (2000) 'The external validity of Asperger Disorder: Lack of evidence from the domain of neuropsychology.' *Journal of Abnormal Psychology 109*, 2, 227–238.

Minshew, N.J., Goldstein, G., Muenz, L.R. and Payton, J.B. (1992) 'Neuropsychological functioning of nonmentally retarded autistic individuals.' *Journal of Clinical and Experimental Neuropsychology 14*, 5, 749–761.

Minshew, N.J., Goldstein, G. and Siegel, D.J. (1997) 'Neuropsychologic functioning in autism: Profile of a complex information processing disorder.' *Journal of the International Neuro- psychological Society 3*, 4, 303–316.

Modahl, C., Green, L., Fein, D., Morris, M., Waterhouse, L., Feinstein, C. and Levin, H. (1998) 'Plasma oxytocin levels in autistic children.' *Biological Psychiatry 43*, 4, 270–277.

Moreno, S. (1992) 'A parent's view of more able people with autism.' In E. Schopler and G.B. Mesibov (eds) *High-functioning Individuals with Autism.* New York: Plenum Press.

Morgan, S.B., Cutrer, P.S., Coplin, J.W. and Rodrigue, J.R. (1989) 'Do autistic children differ from retarded and normal children in Piagetian sensorimotor functioning?' *Journal of Child Psychology and Psychiatry and Allied Disciplines 30*, 6, 857–864.

Mottron, L. (2004) 'Matching strategies in cognitive research with individuals with high-functioning autism: Current practices, instrument biases, and recommendations.' *Journal of Autism and Developmental Disorders 34*, 1, 19–27.

Mottron, L., Burack, J.A., Stauder, J.E.A. and Robaey, P. (1999) 'Perceptual processing among high-functioning persons with autism.' *Journal of Child Psychology and Psychiatry 40*, 2, 203–211.

Mountz, J.M., Tolbert, L.C., Lill, D.W., Katholi, C.R. and Liu, H.G. (1995) 'Functional deficits in autistic disorder: Characterization by technetium-99m-HMPAO and SPECT.' *Journal of Nuclear Medicine 36*, 7, 1156–1162.

Muller, R.A., Behen, M.E., Rothermel, R.D., Chugani, D.C., Muzik, O., Mangner, T.J. and Chugani, H.T. (1999) 'Brain mapping of language and auditory perception in high-functioning autistic adults: A PET study.' *Journal of Autism and Developmental Disorders 29*, 1, 19–31.

Mundy, P. (1995) 'Joint attention and social-emotional approach behavior in children with autism.' *Development and Psychopathology 7*, 1, 63–82.

Mundy, P., Sigman, M. and Kasari, C. (1990) 'A longitudinal study of joint attention and language development in autistic children.' *Journal of Autism and Developmental Disorders 20*, 1, 115–128.

Murch, S.H., Anthony, A., Casson, D.H., Malik, M., Berelowitz, M., Dhillon, A.P., Thomson, M.A., Valentine, A., Davies, S.E. and Walker-Smith, J.A. (2004) 'Retraction of an interpretation.' *Lancet 363*, 9411, 750.

Myles, B.S., Cook, K.T., Miller, N.E., Rinner, L. and Robbins, L.A. (2000) *Asperger Syndrome and Sensory Issues: Practical Solutions for Making Sense of the World.* Shawnee Mission, KS: Autism Asperger Publishing.

Narayan, M., Srinath, S., Anderson, G.M. and Meundi, D.B. (1993) 'Cerebrospinal fluid levels of homovanillic acid and 5–hydroxyindoleacetic acid in autism.' *Biological Psychiatry 33*, 8–9, 630–635.

National Research Council (US) Committee on Educational Interventions for Children with Autism (2001) *Educating Children with Autism.* Washington, DC: National Academy Press.

Nelson, K.B., Grether, J.K., Croen, L.A., Dambrosia, J.M., Dickens, B.F., Jelliffe, L.L., Hansen, R.L. and Phillips, T.M. (2001) 'Neuropeptides and neurotrophins in neonatal blood of children with autism, mental retardation.' *Annals of Neurology 49,* 597–606.

Norman-Bain, J. (1998) *The Autistic Community,* retrieved from http://www.isn.net/~jypsy/community.htm (Janet Norman-Bain's web page).

Novick, B., Vaughan, H.G., Jr., Kurtzberg, D. and Simson, R. (1980) 'An electrophysiologic indication of auditory processing defects in autism.' *Psychiatry Research 3,* 1, 107–114.

Nyden, A., Gillberg, C., Hjelmquist, E. and Heiman, M. (1999) 'Executive function/attention deficits in boys with Asperger syndrome, attention disorder and reading/writing disorder.' *Autism 3,* 3, 213–228.

Oatley, K. (1992) 'Integrative action of narrative.' In D.J. Stein and J.E. Young (eds) *Cognitive Science and Clinical Disorders.* San Diego, CA: Academic Press.

Ohnishi, T., Matsuda, H., Hashimoto, T., Kunihiro, T., Nishikawa, M., Uema, T. and Sasaki, M. (2000) 'Abnormal regional cerebral blood flow in childhood autism.' *Brain 123,* 1838–1844.

O'Riordan, M.A., Plaisted, K.C., Driver, J. and Baron-Cohen, S. (2001) 'Superior visual search in autism.' *Journal of Experimental Psychology: Human Perception and Performance 27,* 3, 719–730.

Osterling, J. and Dawson, G. (1994) 'Early recognition of children with autism: A study of first birthday home videotapes.' *Journal of Autism and Developmental Disorders 24,* 3, 247–257.

Ozonoff, S. (1995) 'Executive functions in autism.' In E. Schopler and G.B. Mesibov (eds) *Learning and Cognition in Autism.* New York: Plenum Press.

Ozonoff, S. and Jensen, J. (1999) 'Brief report: Specific executive function profiles in three neurodevelopmental disorders.' *Journal of Autism and Developmental Disorders 29,* 2, 171–177.

Ozonoff, S. and Miller, J.N. (1995) 'Teaching theory of mind: A new approach to social skills training for individuals with autism.' *Journal of Autism and Developmental Disorders 25,* 4, 415–433.

Ozonoff, S., Pennington, B.F. and Rogers, S.J. (1990) 'Are there emotion perception deficits in young autistic children?' *Journal of Child Psychology and Psychiatry 31,* 3, 343–361.

Ozonoff, S., Pennington, B.F. and Rogers, S.J. (1991) 'Executive function deficits in high- functioning autistic individuals: Relationship to theory of mind.' *Journal of Child Psychology and Psychiatry and Allied Disciplines 32,* 7, 1081–1105.

Ozonoff, S., Rogers, S.J. and Pennington, B.F. (1991) 'Asperger's syndrome: Evidence of an empirical distinction from high-functioning autism.' *Journal of Child Psychology and Psychiatry 32,* 7, 1107–1122.

Ozonoff, S., South, M. and Miller, J.N. (2000) 'DSM-IV-defined Asperger syndrome: Cognitive, behavioral and early history differentiation from high-functioning autism.' *Autism 4,* 1, 29–46.

Ozonoff, S. and Strayer, D.L. (2001) 'Further evidence of intact working memory in autism.' *Journal of Autism and Developmental Disorders 31,* 3, 257–263.

Ozonoff, S., Strayer, D.L., McMahon, W.M. and Filloux, F. (1994) 'Executive function abilities in autism and Tourette syndrome: An information processing approach.' *Journal of Child Psychology and Psychiatry 35,* 6, 1015–1032.

Pascualvaca, D.M., Fantie, B.D., Papageorgiou, M. and Mirsky, A.F. (1998) 'Attentional capacities in children with autism: Is there a general deficit in shifting focus?' *Journal of Autism and Developmental Disorders 28,* 6, 467–478.

Paul, R. (2003) 'Promoting social communication in high functioning individuals with autistic spectrum disorders.' *Child and Adolescent Psychiatric Clinics of North America 12,* 1, 87–106.

Pennington, B.F. and Ozonoff, S. (1996) 'Executive functions and developmental psychopathology.' *Journal of Child Psychology and Psychiatry and Allied Disciplines 37,* 1, 51–87.

Peterson, C.C. and Siegal, M. (1997) 'Domain specificity and everyday biological, physical, and psychological thinking in normal, autistic, and deaf children.' *New Directions for Child Development 75,* 55–70.

Peterson, C.C. and Siegal, M. (2000) 'Insights into theory of mind from deafness and autism.' *Mind and Language 15,* 1, 123–145.

Philippe, A., Guilloud-Bataille, M., Martinez, M., Gillberg, C., Rastam, M., Sponheim, E., Coleman, M., Zappella, M., Aschauer, H., Penet, C., Feingold, J., Brice, A. and Leboyer, M. (2002) 'Analysis of ten candidate genes in autism by association and linkage.' *American Journal of Medical Genetics 114,* 2, 125–128.

Phillips, W., Gomez, J.C., Baron-Cohen, S., Laa, V. and Riviere, A. (1995) 'Treating people as objects, agents, or "subjects": How young children with and without autism make requests.' *Journal of Child Psychology and Psychiatry 36*, 8, 1383–1398.

Pierce, K. and Courchesne, E. (2000) 'Exploring the neurofunctional organization of face processing in autism.' *Archives of General Psychiatry 57*, 4, 344–346.

Pierce, K., Muller, R.A., Ambrose, J., Allen, G. and Courchesne, E. (2001) 'Face processing occurs outside the fusiform "face area" in autism: Evidence from functional MRI.' *Brain 124*, pt 10, 2059–2073.

Pierce, K. and Schreibman, L. (1995) 'Increasing complex social behaviors in children with autism: Effects of peer-implemented pivotal response training.' *Journal of Applied Behavior Analysis 28*, 3, 285–295.

Pierce, K. and Schreibman, L. (1997) 'Multiple peer use of pivotal response training to increase social behaviors of classmates with autism: Results from trained and untrained peers.' *Journal of Applied Behavior Analysis 30*, 1, 157–160.

Piven, J. (1997) 'The biological basis of autism.' *Current Opinion in Neurobiology 7*, 5, 708–712.

Piven, J., Arndt, S., Bailey, J. and Andreasen, N. (1996) 'Regional brain enlargement in autism: A magnetic resonance imaging study.' *Journal of the American Academy of Child and Adolescent Psychiatry 35*, 4, 530–536.

Piven, J., Bailey, J., Ranson, B.J. and Arndt, S. (1997) 'An MRI study of the corpus callosum in autism.' *American Journal of Psychiatry 154*, 8, 1051–1056.

Piven, J., Berthier, M.L., Starkstein, S.E., Nehme, E., Pearlson, G. and Folstein, S. (1990) 'Magnetic resonance imaging evidence for a defect of cerebral cortical development in autism.' *American Journal of Psychiatry 147*, 6, 734–739.

Piven, J., Harper, J., Palmer, P. and Arndt, S. (1996) 'Course of behavioral change in autism: A retrospective study of high-IQ adolescents and adults.' *Journal of the American Academy of Child and Adolescent Psychiatry 35*, 4, 523–529.

Piven, J., Saliba, K., Bailey, J. and Arndt, S. (1997) 'An MRI study of autism: The cerebellum revisited.' *Neurology 49*, 2, 546–551.

Piven, J., Simon, J., Chase, G.A., Wzorek, M., Landa, R., Gayle, J. and Folstein, S. (1993) 'The etiology of autism: Pre-, peri- and neonatal factors.' *Journal of the American Academy of Child and Adolescent Psychiatry 32*, 6, 1256–1263.

Plaisted, K., O'Riordan, M. and Baron-Cohen, S. (1998) 'Enhanced visual search for a conjunctive target in autism: A research note.' *Journal of Child Psychology and Psychiatry 39*, 5, 777–783.

Plaisted, K., Swettenham, J. and Rees, L. (1999) 'Children with autism show local precedence in a divided attention task and global precedence in a selective attention task.' *Journal of Child Psychology and Psychiatry 40*, 5, 733–742.

Policastro, E. and Gardner, H. (1999) 'From case studies to robust generalizations: An approach to the study of creativity.' In R.J. Sternberg (ed.) *Handbook of Creativity*. New York, NY: Cambridge University Press.

Polich, J. and Kok, A. (1995) 'Cognitive and biological determinants of P300: An integrative review.' *Biological Psychology 41*, 2, 103–146.

Polkinghorne, D. (1988) *Narrative Knowing and the Human Sciences*. Albany: State University of New York Press.

Premack, D. and Woodruff, G. (1978) 'Does the chimpanzee have a theory of mind? *Behavioural and Brain Sciences 1*, 516–526.

Prior, M.R. (2003) *Learning and Behavior Problems in Asperger Syndrome*. New York: Guilford Press.

Quill, K.A. (ed.) (1995) *Teaching Children with Autism: Strategies to Enhance Communication and Socialization*. New York: Delmar.

Raichle, M.E. (2003) 'Functional brain imaging and human brain function.' *Journal of Neuroscience 23*, 10, 3959–3962.

Renner, P., Klinger, L.G. and Klinger, M.R. (2000) 'Implicit and explicit memory in autism: Is autism an amnesic disorder?' *Journal of Autism and Developmental Disorders 30*, 1, 3–14.

Richters, J.E. (1997) 'The Hubble hypothesis and the developmentalist's dilemma.' *Development and Psychopathology 9*, 2, 193–229.

Ricoeur, P. (1987) *Time and Narrative* (vol. 3, trans. K. Blamey and D. Pellauer). Chicago: University of Chicago Press.

Rieffe, C., Meerum Terwogt, M. and Stockmann, L. (2000) 'Understanding atypical emotions among children with autism.' *Journal of Autism and Developmental Disorders 30*, 3, 195–203.

Rimland, B. (1964) *Infantile Autism: The Syndrome and its Implications for a Neural Theory of Behavior.* New York: Appleton-Century-Crofts.

Rincover, A. and Ducharme, J.M. (1987) 'Variables influencing stimulus overselectivity and "tunnel vision" in developmentally delayed children.' *American Journal of Mental Deficiency 91,* 4, 422–430.

Rinehart, N.J., Bradshaw, J.L., Moss, S.A., Brereton, A.V. and Tonge, B.J. (2000) 'Atypical interference of local detail on global processing in high-functioning autism and Asperger's disorder.' *Journal of Child Psychology and Psychiatry 41,* 6, 769–778.

Rinehart, N.J., Bradshaw, J.L., Moss, S.A., Brereton, A.V. and Tonge, B.J. (2001) 'A deficit in shifting attention present in high-functioning autism but not Asperger's disorder.' *Autism 5,* 1, 67–80.

Ritvo, E.R., Yuwiler, A., Geller, E., Ornitz, E.M., Saeger, K. and Plotkin, S. (1970) 'Increased blood serotonin and platelets in early infantile autism.' *Archives of General Psychiatry 23,* 6, 566–572.

Rodgers, J. (2000) 'Visual perception and Asperger syndrome: Central coherence deficit or hierarchization deficit? A pilot study.' *Autism 4,* 3, 321–329.

Rodier, P.M. (2000) 'The early origins of autism.' *Scientific American 282,* 2, 56–63.

Rodier, P.M. (2004) '2003 Warkany Lecture: Autism as a birth defect.' *Birth Defects Research (Part A): Clinical and Molecular Teratology 70,* 1, 1–6.

Rodier, P.M. and Hyman, S.L. (1998) 'Early environmental factors in autism.' *Mental Retardation and Developmental Disabilities Research Reviews 4,* 2, 121–128.

Rogers, S.J. (2000) 'Interventions that facilitate socialization in children with autism.' *Journal of Autism and Developmental Disorders 30,* 5, 399–409.

Rogers, S.J., Hepburn, S.L., Stackhouse, T. and Wehner, E. (2003) 'Imitation performance in toddlers with autism and those with other developmental disorders.' *Journal of Child Psychology and Psychiatry 44,* 5, 763–781.

Rogers, S.J., Ozonoff, S. and Maslin-Cole, C. (1991) 'A comparative study of attachment behavior in young children with autism or other psychiatric disorders.' *Journal of the American Academy of Child and Adolescent Psychiatry 30,* 3, 483–488.

Rogers, S.J., Ozonoff, S. and Maslin-Cole, C. (1993) 'Developmental aspects of attachment behavior in young children with pervasive developmental disorders.' *Journal of the American Academy of Child and Adolescent Psychiatry 32,* 6, 1274–1282.

Rogers, S.J. and Pennington, B.F. (1991) 'A theoretical approach to the deficits in infantile autism.' *Development and Psychopathology 3,* 137–162.

Rourke, B.P. (1995) *Syndrome of Nonverbal Learning Disabilities: Neurodevelopmental Manifestations.* New York: Guilford Press.

Rourke, B.P., del Dotto, J.E., Rourke, S.B. and Casey, J.E. (1990) 'Nonverbal Learning Disabilities: The Syndrome and a Case Study.' *Journal of School Psychology 28,* 4, 361–385.

Rourke, B.P. and Tsatsanis, K.D. (2000) 'Nonverbal learning disabilities and Asperger syndrome.' In A. Klin, F.R. Volkmar and S.S. Sparrow (eds) *Asperger Syndrome.* New York: Guilford Press.

Rowe, C.C., Berkovic, S.F., Austin, M.C., Saling, M., Kalnins, R.M., McKay, W.J. and Bladin, P.F. (1991) 'Visual and quantitative analysis of interictal SPECT with technetium-99m-HMPAO in temporal lobe epilepsy.' *Journal of Nuclear Medicine 32,* 9, 1688–1694.

Ruble, L.A. and Scott, M.M. (2002) 'Executive functions and the natural habitat behaviors of children with autism.' *Autism 6,* 4, 365–381.

Russell, J. (1997) 'How executive disorders can bring about an inadequate "theory of mind".' In J. Russell (ed.) *Autism as an Executive Disorder.* Oxford, UK: Oxford University Press.

Russell, J. and Hill, E.L. (2001) 'Action-monitoring and intention reporting in children with autism.' *Journal of Child Psychology and Psychiatry and Allied Disciplines 42,* 3, 317–328.

Russell, J., Jarrold, C. and Hood, B. (1999) 'Two intact executive capacities in children with autism: Implications for the core executive dysfunctions in the disorder.' *Journal of Autism and Developmental Disorders 29,* 2, 103–112.

Russell, J., Mauthner, N., Sharpe, S. and Tidswell, T. (1991) 'The windows task as a measure of strategic deception in preschoolers and autistic subjects.' *British Journal of Developmental Psychology 9,* 331–349.

Rutter, M. (1978) 'Language disorder and infantile autism.' In M. Rutter and E. Schopler (eds) *Autism: A Reappraisal of Concepts and Treatment.* New York: Plenum Press.

Rutter, M., Greenfeld, D. and Lockyer, L. (1967) 'A 5 to 15 year follow-up study of infantile psychosis. II. Social and behavioural outcome.' *British Journal of Psychiatry 113,* 504, 1183–1199.

Rutter, M., Bailey, A., Bolton, P. and Le Couteur, A. (1994) 'Autism and known medical conditions: Myth and substance.' *Journal of Child Psychology and Psychiatry and Allied Disciplines 35,* 2, 311–322.

Ryu, Y.H., Lee, J.D., Yoon, P.H., Kim, D.I., Lee, H.B. and Shin, Y.J. (1999) 'Perfusion impairments in infantile autism on technetium-99m ethyl cysteinate dimer brain single-photon emission tomography: Comparison with findings on magnetic resonance imaging.' *European Journal of Nuclear Medicine and Molecular Imaging 26*, 3, 253–259.

Sacks, O. (1987) *The Man who Mistook his Wife for a Hat.* New York: Harper.

Sacks, O. (1996) *An Anthropologist on Mars.* Toronto: Vintage Canada.

Sandberg, A.D., Nyden, A., Gillberg, C. and Hjelmquist, E. (1993) 'The cognitive profile in infantile autism: A study of 70 children and adolescents using the Griffiths Mental Development Scale.' *British Journal of Psychology 84*, 3, 365–373.

Sarrias, M.J., Cabre, P., Martinez, E. and Artigas, F. (1990) 'Relationship between serotoninergic measures in blood and cerebrospinal fluid simultaneously obtained in humans.' *Journal of Neurochemistry 54*, 3, 783–786.

Sattler, J.M. (1992) *Assessment of Children* (3rd edn). San Diego, CA: Jerome M. Sattler.

Schain, R.J. and Freedman, D.X. (1961) 'Studies on 5–hydroxyindole metabolism in autistic and other mentally retarded children.' *Journal of Pediatrics 58*, 315–320.

Schneider, E. (1999) *Discovering My Autism: Apologia Pro Vita Sua (with apologies to Cardinal Newman).* London: Jessica Kingsley Publishers.

Schopler, E. (1996) 'Are autism and Asperger syndrome (AS) different labels or different disabilities?' *Journal of Autism and Developmental Disorders 26*, 1, 109–110.

Schopler, E. (1998) 'Premature popularization of Asperger syndrome.' In E. Schopler, G.B. Mesibov and L.J. Kunce (eds) *Asperger Syndrome or High Functioning Autism?* New York: Plenum Press.

Schultz, R.T., Gauthier, I., Klin, A., Fulbright, R.K., Anderson, A.W., Volkmar, F., Skudlarski, P., Lacadie, C., Cohen, D.J. and Gore, J.C. (2000) 'Abnormal ventral temporal cortical activity during face discrimination among individuals with autism and Asperger syndrome.' *Archives of General Psychiatry 57*, 4, 331–340.

Sears, L.L., Vest, C., Mohamed, S., Bailey, J., Ranson, B.J. and Piven, J. (1999) 'An MRI study of the basal ganglia in autism.' *Progress in Neuro-Psychopharmacology and Biological Psychiatry 23*, 4, 613–624.

Shah, A. and Frith, U. (1993) 'Why do autistic individuals show superior performance on the block design task?' *Journal of Child Psychology and Psychiatry 34*, 8, 1351–1364.

Sigman, M., Kasari, C., Kwon, J.H. and Yirmiya, N. (1992) 'Responses to the negative emotions of others by autistic, mentally-retarded, and normal-children.' *Child Development 63*, 4, 796–807.

Sigman, M. and Mundy, P. (1989) 'Social attachments in autistic children.' *Journal of the American Academy of Child and Adolescent Psychiatry 28*, 1, 74–81.

Sigman, M. and Ungerer, J.A. (1984) 'Attachment behaviors in autistic children.' *Journal of Autism and Developmental Disorders 14*, 3, 231–244.

Sinclair, J. (1992) 'Bridging the gaps: An inside-out view of autism (Or, do you know what I don't know?)'. In E. Schopler and G.B. Mesibov (eds) *High-functioning Individuals with Autism.* New York: Plenum Press.

Sinclair, J. (1993) 'Don't mourn for us.' Retrieved February 23, 2004, from http://web.syr.edu/~jisincla/dontmourn.htm (original work published in 1993 in *Our Voice*, [the newsletter of Autism Network International] *1*, 3).

Smith, I.M. (2000) 'Motor functioning in Asperger syndrome.' In A. Klin, F.R. Volkmar and S.S. Sparrow (eds) *Asperger Syndrome.* New York: Guilford Press.

Smith, I.M. and Bryson, S.E. (1994) 'Imitation and action in autism: A critical review.' *Psychological Bulletin 116*, 2, 259–273.

Sojkova, J., Lewis, P.J., Siegel, A.H., Siegel, A.M., Roberts, D.W., Thadani, V.M. and Williamson, P.D. (2003) 'Does asymmetric basal ganglia or thalamic activation aid in seizure foci lateralization on ictal SPECT studies?' *Journal of Nuclear Medicine 44*, 9, 1379–1386.

Sparks, B.F., Friedman, S.D., Shaw, D.W., Aylward, E.H., Echelard, D., Artru, A.A., Maravilla, K.R., Giedd, J.N., Munson, J., Dawson, G. and Dager, S.R. (2002) 'Brain structural abnormalities in young children with autism spectrum disorder.' *Neurology 59*, 2, 184–192.

Stahl, S.M., Woo, D.J., Mefford, I.N., Berger, P.A. and Ciaranello, R.D. (1983) 'Hyperserotonemia and platelet serotonin uptake and release in schizophrenia and affective disorders.' *American Journal of Psychiatry 140*, 1, 26–30.

Stake, R.E. (1995) *The Art of Case Study Research.* Thousand Oaks, CA: Sage Publications.

Stake, R.E. (2000) 'Case studies.' In N.K. Denzin and Y.S. Lincoln (eds) *Handbook of Qualitative Research.* Thousand Oaks, CA: Sage Publications.

Starkstein, S.E., Vazquez, S., Vrancic, D., Nanclares, V., Manes, F., Piven, J. and Plebst, C. (2000) 'SPECT findings in mentally retarded autistic individuals.' *Journal of Neuropsychiatry and Clinical Neurosciences 12*, 3, 370–375.

Sternberg, R.J. (1986) *Beyond IQ: A Triarchic Theory of Human Intelligence.* Cambridge: Cambridge University Press.

Sternberg, R.J. (1997) *Successful Intelligence.* New York: Plume.

Sternberg, R.J. (2000) 'The concept of intelligence.' In R.J. Sternberg (ed.) *Handbook of Human Intelligence.* New York: Cambridge.

Sternberg, R.J., Grigorenko, E.L. and Bundy, D.A. (2001) 'The predictive value of IQ.' *Merrill-Palmer Quarterly 47*, 1, 1–41.

Sternberg, R.J. and Wagner, R.K. (1994) *Mind in Context: Interactionist Perspectives on Human Intelligence.* Cambridge: Cambridge University Press.

Stone, W.L. and Caro-Martinez, L.M. (1990) 'Naturalistic observations of spontaneous com- munication in autistic children.' *Journal of Autism and Developmental Disorders 20*, 4, 437–453.

Strawn, J.R., Ekhator, N.N., Anthenelli, R.M., Baker, D.G., Maxwell, R.A., Hill, K.K. and Geracioti, T.D. (2002) 'Intra- and inter-individual relationships between central and peripheral serotonergic activity in humans: A serial cerebrospinal fluid sampling study.' *Life Sciences 71*, 10, 1219–1225.

Szatmari, P. (2000) 'The classification of autism, Asperger's syndrome and pervasive developmental disorder.' *Canadian Journal of Psychiatry 45*, 8, 731–738.

Szatmari, P., Tuff, L., Finlayson, M.A. and Bartolucci, G. (1990) 'Asperger's syndrome and autism: Neurocognitive aspects.' *Journal of the American Academy of Child and Adolescent Psychiatry 29*, 1, 130–136.

Tager-Flusberg, H. (2001a) 'A re-examination of the theory of mind hypothesis of autism.' In J.A. Burack, T. Charman, N. Yirmiya and P.R. Zelazo (eds) *The Development of Autism: Perspectives from Theory and Research.* Mahwah, NJ: Lawrence Erlbaum.

Tager-Flusberg, H. (2001b) 'Understanding the language and communicative impairments in autism.' *International Review of Research in Mental Retardation 23*, 185–205.

Tan, J. and Harris, P.L. (1991) 'Autistic children understand seeing and wanting.' *Development and Psychopathology 3*, 2, 163–174.

Tanguay, P.E. (2000) 'Pervasive developmental disorders: A 10-year review.' *Journal of the American Academy of Child and Adolescent Psychiatry 39*, 9, 1079–1095.

Tantam, D. (1991) 'Asperger syndrome in adulthood.' In U. Frith (ed.) *Autism and Asperger Syndrome.* New York: Cambridge University Press.

Tantam, D. (2000) 'Psychological disorder in adolescents and adults with Asperger syndrome.' *Autism 4*, 1, 47–62.

Tantam, D. (2003) 'The challenge of adolescents and adults with Asperger syndromes.' *Child and Adolescent Psychiatric Clinics of North America 12*, 1, 143–163.

Tarr, M.J. and Cheng, Y.D. (2003) 'Learning to see faces and objects.' *Trends in Cognitive Sciences 7*, 1, 23–30.

Tarr, M.J. and Gauthier, I. (2000) 'FFA: A flexible fusiform area for subordinate-level visual processing automatized by expertise.' *Nature Neuroscience 3*, 8, 764–769.

Taylor, C. (1989) *Sources of the Self: The Making of the Modern Identity.* Cambridge, MA: Harvard University Press.

Taylor, S.E. and Brown, J.D. (1988) 'Illusion and well-being: A social psychological perspective on mental-health.' *Psychological Bulletin 103*, 2, 193–210.

Tentler, D., Johannesson, T., Johansson, M., Rastam, M., Gillberg, C., Orsmark, C., Carlsson, B., Wahlstrom, J. and Dahl, N. (2003) 'A candidate region for Asperger syndrome defined by two 17p breakpoints.' *European Journal of Human Genetics 11*, 2, 189–195.

Thelen, E. and Smith, L.B. (1994) *A Dynamic Systems Approach to the Development of Cognition and Action.* Cambridge, MA: MIT Press.

Toichi, M. and Kamio, Y. (2002) 'Long-term memory and levels-of-processing in autism.' *Neuropsychologia 40*, 7, 964–969.

Tonge, B.J., Brereton, A.V., Gray, K.M. and Einfeld, S.L. (1999) 'Behavioural and emotional disturbance in high-functioning autism and Asperger syndrome.' *Autism 3*, 2, 117–130.

Toomey, J. and Adams, L.A. (1995) 'Naturalistic observation of children with autism: Evidence for intersubjectivity.' *New Directions for Child Development 69*, 75–89.

Townsend, J., Harris, N.S. and Courchesne, E. (1996) 'Visual attention abnormalities in autism: Delayed orienting to location.' *Journal of the International Neuropsychological Society 2*, 6, 541–550.
Townsend, J., Westerfield, M., Leaver, E., Makeig, S., Jung, T.-P., Pierce, K. and Courchesne, E. (2001) 'Event-related brain response abnormalities in autism: Evidence for impaired cerebello-frontal spatial attention networks.' *Cognitive Brain Research 11*, 1, 127–145.
Trevarthen, C., Aitken, K., Papoudi, D. and Robarts, J. (1998) *Children with Autism: Diagnosis and Interventions to Meet their Needs.* London: Jessica Kingsley Publishers.
Tsai, L.Y. (1999) 'Psychopharmacology in autism.' *Psychosomatic Medicine 61*, 5, 651–665.
Tsatsanis, K.D. (2003) 'Outcome research in Asperger syndrome and autism.' *Child and Adolescent Psychiatric Clinics of North America 12*, 1, 47–63.
Tuchman, R. and Rapin, I. (2002) 'Epilepsy in autism.' *The Lancet Neurology 1*, 6, 352–358.
Twachtman Cullen, D. (1998) 'Language and communication in high-functioning autism and Asperger syndrome.' In E. Schopler, G.B. Mesibov and L.J. Kunce (eds) *Asperger Syndrome or High Functioning Autism?* New York: Plenum Press.
Uttal, W.R. (2001) *The New Phrenology. The Limits of Localizing Cognitive Processes in the Brain.* Cambridge, MA: MIT Press.
Veenstra-Vanderweele, J. and Cook, E., Jr (2003) 'Genetics of childhood disorders: XLVI. Autism, part 5: Genetics of autism.' *Journal of the American Academy of Child and Adolescent Psychiatry 42*, 1, 116–118.
Verbaten, M.N., Roelofs, J.W., Van Engeland, H., Kenemans, J.K. and Slangen, J.L. (1991) 'Abnormal visual event-related potentials of autistic children.' *Journal of Autism and Developmental Disorders 21*, 4, 449–470.
Volkmar, F.R. (2001) 'Pharmacological interventions in autism: Theoretical and practical issues.' *Journal of Clinical Child Psychology 30*, 1, 80–87.
Volkmar, F.R. and Cohen, D.J. (1985) 'The experience of infantile autism: A first-person account by Tony W.' *Journal of Autism and Developmental Disorders 15*, 1, 47–54.
Volkmar, F.R. and Klin, A. (2000) 'Diagnostic issues in Asperger syndrome.' In A. Klin, F.R. Volkmar and S.S. Sparrow (eds) *Asperger Syndrome.* New York: Guilford Press.
Volkmar, F.R., d, R. (2000) 'Asperger's disorder.' *American Journal of Psychiatry 157*, 2, 262–267.
Volkmar, F.R., Lord, C., Bailey, A., Schultz, R.T. and Klin, A. (2004) 'Autism and pervasive developmental disorders.' *Journal of Child Psychology and Psychiatry 45*, 1, 135–170.
Vygotsky, L.S. (1934/1986) *Thought and Language* (trans. A. Kozulin). Cambridge, MA: MIT Press.
Vygotsky, L.S., Rieber, R.W. and Carton, A.S. (1924/1993) *The Collected Works of L.S. Vygotsky, Vol. 2: The Fundamentals of Defectology* (trans. J.E. Knox and C.B. Stevens). New York: Plenum Press. (Original work published between 1924 and 1932.)
Wakefield, A.J., Murch, S.H., Anthony, A., Linnell, J., Casson, D.M., Malik, M., Berelowitz, M., Dhillon, A.P., Thomson, M.A., Harvey, P., Valentine, A., Davies, S.E. and Walker-Smith, J.A. (1998) 'Ileal-lymphoid-nodular hyperplasia, non-specific colitis, and pervasive developmental disorder in children.' *Lancet 351*, 9103, 637–641.
Wheelwright, S. and Baron-Cohen, S. (2001) 'The link between autism and skills such as engineering, maths, physics and computing: A reply to Jarrold and Routh.' *Autism 5*, 2, 223–227.
Whitaker, P., Barratt, P., Joy, H., Potter, M. and Thomas, G. (1998) 'Children with autism and peer group support: Using "Circle of friends".' *British Journal of Special Education 25*, 2, 60–64.
Williams, D. (1996a) *Autism, an Inside-out Approach: An Innovative Look at the Mechanics of 'autism' and its Developmental 'Cousins'.* London: Jessica Kingsley Publishers.
Williams, D. (1996b) *Like Color to the Blind: Soul Searching and Soul Finding.* New York: Times Books.
Williams, D. (1998) *Autism and Sensing: The Unlost Instinct.* London: Jessica Kingsley Publishers.
Williams, D. (1999a) *Nobody Nowhere: The Extraordinary Autobiography of an Autistic.* London: Jessica Kingsley Publishers.
Williams, D. (1999b) *Somebody Somewhere: Breaking Free from the World of Autism.* London: Jessica Kingsley Publishers.
Wilson, T.D. and Dunn, E.W. (2004) 'Self-knowledge: Its limits, value, and potential for improvement.' *Annual Review of Psychology 55*, 1, 493–518.
Wing, L. (1981) 'Asperger syndrome: A clinical account.' *Psychological Medicine 11*, 115–129.
Wing, L. (1988) 'The continuum of autistic characteristics.' In E. Schopler and G.B. Mesibov (eds) *Diagnosis and Assessment in Autism.* New York: Plenum Press.
Wing, L. (1991) 'The relationship between Asperger's syndrome and Kanner's autism.' In U. Frith (ed.) *Autism and Asperger Syndrome.* Cambridge: Cambridge University Press.

Wing, L. (2000) 'Past and future of research on Asperger syndrome.' In A. Klin, F.R. Volkmar and S.S. Sparrow (eds) *Asperger Syndrome.* New York: Guilford Press.

Winner, E. (1996) *Gifted Children: Myths and Realities.* New York: Basic Books.

Winner, E. (1998) 'Uncommon talents: Gifted children, prodigies and savants.' *Scientific American 9,* 4, 32–37.

Wolff, S. (1996) 'The first account of the syndrome Asperger described?' *European Child and Adolescent Psychiatry 5,* 3, 119–132.

World Health Organization (WHO) (1992) *The ICD-10 Classification of Mental and Behavioral Disorders.* Geneva: World Health Organization.

Yang, P.C., Lee, B.F., Hsu, H.Y. and Jong, Y.J. (2001) 'Technetium-99m HMPAO SPECT for children with developmental language disorder.' *NeuroImage 13,* 6, S631–S631.

Yewchuk, C. and Lupart, J.L. (2000) 'Inclusive education for gifted students with disabilities.' In K.A. Heller, F.J. Moenks, R. Sternberg and R. Subotnik (eds) *International Handbook of Research and Development of Giftedness and Talent* (2nd edn). Amsterdam: Pergamon.

Yin, R.K. (1989) *Case Study Research: Design and Methods* (rev. edn). Newbury Park, CA: Sage.

Yirmiya, N., Sigman, M.D., Kasari, C. and Mundy, P. (1992) 'Empathy and cognition in high-functioning children with autism.' *Child Development 63,* 1, 150–160.

Yirmiya, N., Solomonica-Levi, D., Shulman, C. and Pilowsky, T. (1996) 'Theory of mind abilities in individuals with autism, Down syndrome, and mental retardation of unknown etiology: The role of age and intelligence.' *Journal of Child Psychology and Psychiatry 37,* 8, 1003–1014.

Ylisaukko-oja, T., Nieminen-von Wendt, T., Kempas, E., Sarenius, S., Varilo, T., von Wendt, L., Peltonen, L. and Jarvela, I. (2004) 'Genome-wide scan for loci of Asperger syndrome.' *Molecular Psychiatry 9,* 2, 161–168.

Yonan, A.L., Alarcon, M., Cheng, R., Magnusson, P.K., Spence, S.J., Palmer, A.A., Grunn, A., Juo, S.H., Terwilliger, J.D., Liu, J., Cantor, R.M., Geschwind, D.H. and Gilliam, T.C. (2003) 'A genomewide screen of 345 families for autism-susceptibility loci.' *American Journal of Medical Genetics 73,* 4, 886–897.

Yule, W. (1978) 'Research methodology: What are the "correct controls"?' In M. Rutter and E. Schopler (eds) *Autism: A Reappraisal of Concepts and Treatment.* New York: Plenum Press.

Yuwiler, A., Shih, J.C., Chen, C.H., Ritvo, E.R., Hanna, G., Ellison, G.W. and King, B.H. (1992) 'Hyperserotoninemia and antiserotonin antibodies in autism and other disorders.' *Journal of Autism and Developmental Disorders 22,* 1, 33–45.

Zelazo, P.D., Burack, J.A., Benedetto, E. and Frye, D. (1996) 'Theory of mind and rule use in individuals with Down's syndrome: A test of the uniqueness and specificity claims.' *Journal of Child Psychology and Psychiatry 37,* 4, 479–484.

Zilbovicius, M., Boddaert, N., Belin, P., Poline, J.B., Remy, P., Mangin, J.F., Thivard, L., Barthelemy, C. and Samson, Y. (2000) 'Temporal lobe dysfunction in childhood autism: A PET study.' *American Journal of Psychiatry 157,* 12, 1988–1993.

Zilbovicius, M., Garreau, B., Samson, Y., Remy, P., Barthelemy, C., Syrota, A. and Lelord, G. (1995) 'Delayed maturation of the frontal cortex in childhood autism.' *American Journal of Psychiatry 152,* 2, 248–252.

Zilbovicius, M., Garreau, B., Tzourio, N., Mazoyer, B., Bruck, B., Martinot, J.L., Raynaud, C., Samson, Y., Syrota, A. and Lelord, G. (1992) 'Regional cerebral blood flow in childhood autism: A SPECT study.' *American Journal of Psychiatry 149,* 7, 924–930.

Subject Index

References followed by 'n' indicate notes, with the note number in brackets.

Author Index

References followed by 'n' indicate notes, with the note number in brackets.